Health Systems in Transition: Canada

Written by
Gregory P. Marchildon

Edited by
Sara Allin
Elias Mossialos

University of Toronto Press
Toronto Buffalo London

2005

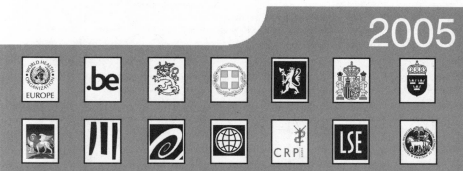

The European Observatory on Health Systems and Policies is a partnership between the World Health Organization Regional Office for Europe, the governments of Belgium, Finland, Greece, Norway, Spain and Sweden, the Veneto Region of Italy, the European Investment Bank, the Open Society Institute, the World Bank, CRP-Santé Luxembourg, the London School of Economics and Political Science, and the London School of Hygiene & Tropical Medicine.

Published by the WHO Regional Office for Europe on behalf of the European Observatory on Health Systems and Policies under the title *Health Systems in Transition: Canada*

The Director of the Regional Office for Europe of the World Health Organization has granted reproduction rights to University of Toronto Press

Published in North America by University of Toronto Press Incorporated, 2006.
Toronto Buffalo London
Printed in Canada

ISBN 13: 978-0-8020-9400-1
ISBN 10: 0-8020-9400-7

∞

Printed on acid-free paper
A catalogue record for this book is available from the University of Toronto Press

University of Toronto Press acknowledges the financial assistance to its publishing program of the Canada Council for the Arts and the Ontario Arts Council.

University of Toronto Press acknowledges the financial support for its publishing activities of the Government of Canada through the Book Publishing Industry Development Program (BPIDP).

Contents

Foreword v

Preface.. vii

Acknowledgements.. ix

Executive summary... xi

1. Introduction.. 1

    1.1 Overview of the health system.. 1

    1.2 Geography and sociodemography 2

    1.3 Economic context 7

    1.4 Political context 8

    1.5 Health status... 12

2. Organizational structure... 19

    2.1 Historical background.. 19

    2.2 Organizational overview 25

    2.3 Patient rights, empowerment and satisfaction 37

3. Financial resources.. 39

    3.1 Revenue collection.. 39

    3.2 Population coverage and basis for entitlement 49

    3.3 Pooling agencies and mechanisms for allocating funds 50

    3.4 Purchaser and purchaser–provider relations 51

    3.5 Payment mechanisms... 52

    3.6 Health care expenditures.. 54

4. Regulation and planning 61

    4.1 Regulation.. 61

    4.2 Planning and health information management 67

5. Physical and human resources 73
   5.1 Physical resources 73
   5.2 Human resources: trends, training, planning and
       registration/licensing 81
6. Provision of services 89
   6.1 Public health 89
   6.2 Patient pathways 92
   6.3 Primary/ambulatory care 93
   6.4 Secondary/inpatient and specialized ambulatory care 95
   6.5 Pharmaceutical care 97
   6.6 Rehabilitation/intermediate care 98
   6.7 Long-term care, home care and other community care 98
   6.8 Services for informal caregivers 99
   6.9 Palliative care 100
   6.10 Mental health care 101
   6.11 Dental health care 101
   6.12 Complementary and alternative health products and services 102
   6.13 Maternal and child health care 103
   6.14 Health care and Aboriginal Canadians 103
7. Principal health care reforms 105
   7.1 Analysis of recent reforms 105
   7.2 Phase one of health reforms, 1988 to 1996 106
   7.3 Phase two of health reforms, 1997 to present 111
8. Assessment of the health system 119
   8.1 Assessing the components: public, mixed and private 119
   8.2 Assessing the public (Medicare) health sector 121
   8.3 Beyond Medicare: assessing the mixed health sector 125
   8.4 Assessing the private health sector 125
   8.5 Overall health status and health indicator performance 126
9. Conclusions 131
10. References 135
11. Useful websites 151

Foreword

All voyages of discovery must necessarily begin with a deeper understanding of one's own self and circumstances. The challenge of understanding health policy and health systems follows the same sound principle.

Claims about all health systems are hotly contested among payers, providers and, increasingly, citizens and patients. It is of considerable value if participants in the policy process have information through an excellent comparative description upon which to base their views. At a minimum this raises the level of debate to a more thoughtful plane. That is what the European Observatory on Health Systems and Policies series has provided in an overall comparative sense. Now Canada is well served by a clear and extremely thorough description of its health system in this monograph authored by Professor Gregory Marchildon, a careful and thoughtful academic and former senior public servant.

One of the most promising developments in Canadian health policy has been the rapid growth of capacity for health services policy work across the nation. Many health research institutes and health policy organizations have been established over the past decade.

Learning about health systems across borders is a tricky business. Often elements of systems seem similar and therefore policy or programme innovations seem transportable. However, without a deeper and more comprehensive understanding the real dynamics and values underlying health systems can be missed, rendering policy innovations imported from elsewhere ineffective or complete failures.

The richness and diversity of the European experience in health policy and health reform should be of enormous relevance to Canadian policy-makers and to Canadians. Without a thorough description of our own system it is not readily apparent how Europeans can easily or insightfully comment. Both the Romanow Royal Commission and the Senate Committee chaired by Senator Michael Kirby looked east across the Atlantic rather than south to the United States. In future such conversations will be aided significantly by the work contained in this paper. Perhaps the Supreme Court of Canada, when it next turns its attention to health and the Charter of Rights, will consider this thoughtful document.

To advance health policy, Canada needs to mine the rich diversity of its varied provincial experiences – ten natural experiments. It also needs to learn about the experience of the nations of Europe, most of which have embedded values similar to Canada in the core of their approach to health service insurance and provision. This profile adds a valuable and high quality asset to the growing body of Canadian analysis of our health system.

Michael B. Decter
Chair, Health Council of Canada
August 2005

Preface

The Health Systems in Transition profiles are country-based reports that provide a detailed description of a health system and of reform and policy initiatives in progress or under development in a specific country. Each profile is produced by country experts in collaboration with the Observatory's research directors and staff. In order to facilitate comparisons between countries, the profiles are based on a template, which is revised periodically. The template provides detailed guidelines and specific questions, definitions and examples needed to compile a profile.

Health Systems in Transition profiles seek to provide relevant information to support policy-makers and analysts in the development of health systems in Europe. They are building blocks that can be used:

- to learn in detail about different approaches to the organization, financing and delivery of health services and the role of the main actors in health systems;
- to describe the institutional framework, the process, content and implementation of health care reform programmes;
- to highlight challenges and areas that require more in-depth analysis; and
- to provide a tool for the dissemination of information on health systems and the exchange of experiences of reform strategies between policy-makers and analysts in different countries.

Compiling the profiles poses a number of methodological problems. In many countries, there is relatively little information available on the health system and the impact of reforms. Due to the lack of a uniform data source, quantitative data on health services are based on a number of different sources, including the WHO Regional Office for Europe health for all database, national statistical offices, Eurostat, the Organisation for Economic Co-operation and Development (OECD) health data, the International Monetary Fund (IMF), the World Bank, and any other relevant sources considered useful by the authors. Data collection methods and definitions sometimes vary, but typically are consistent within each separate series.

A standardized profile has certain disadvantages because the financing and delivery of health care differs across countries. However, it also offers advantages, because it raises similar issues and questions. The Health Systems in Transition profiles can be used to inform policy-makers about experiences in other countries that may be relevant to their own national situation. They can also be used to inform comparative analysis of health systems. This series is an ongoing initiative and material is updated at regular intervals. Comments and suggestions for the further development and improvement of the Health Systems in Transition series are most welcome and can be sent to observatory@who.dk.

Health Systems in Transition profiles and Health Systems in Transition summaries are available on the Observatory's website at www.observatory.dk. A glossary of terms used in the profiles can be found at the following website: www.euro.who.int/observatory/Glossary/Toppage.

Acknowledgements

The Canadian Health System profile was written by Gregory Marchildon (University of Regina). It was edited by Sara Allin (European Observatory on Health Systems and Policies) and Elias Mossialos (European Observatory on Health Systems and Policies). The Research Director for the Canadian Health System profile was Elias Mossialos.

The European Observatory on Health Systems and Policies is especially grateful to Robert Evans, Armine Yalnizyan and Gary Catlin for reviewing the report and for their important contributions.

The author would like to thank the many individuals who have helped in the preparation of this report. The author greatly benefited from the detailed comments, suggestions and information provided by Geoff Ballinger (Canadian Institute for Health Information), Tim Caulfield (University of Alberta), Tony Culyer (Institute for Work and Health and University of York), Donna Magnusson (Saskatchewan Health), Tom McIntosh (Canadian Policy Research Networks), John Richards (Simon Fraser University and C.D. Howe Institute), James Smythe (University of Alberta) and Laurie Thompson (independent health consultant). The author was particularly appreciative of the extensive commentary provided by Robert Evans, Professor of Economics at the University of British Columbia, and the review provided by Pierre-Gerlier Forest, the G.D.W. Cameron Chair and Acting Chief Scientist at Health Canada. They both went far beyond the call of duty in terms of time and effort. In accordance with Observatory protocol, the manuscript was reviewed by Health Canada and the author benefited greatly from the review provided by the Health Policy Branch (Meena Ballantyne, Mary Gregory, and David Lee, assisted by Demetrios Angelis, Jamil Aouiti, Jennifer Cavasin, Roger Guillemette, Paul Kasimatis, Stephen Leclair, Brenda Lipsett, Georgia Livadiotakis, Steven Schwendt, Aruna Sehgal, and Barbara Woodward), the First Nations and Inuit Health Branch (Ian McGrath) and the Corporate

Services Branch (Colleen Bolger and Ross Hodgins) of Health Canada as well as the Public Health Agency of Canada. None of these individuals or organizations is responsible for the author's interpretation or any remaining errors.

From the beginning, Kevin O'Fee's statistical research has been invaluable as well as his assistance as a liaison with Statistics Canada and the Canadian Institutes of Health Research. Nathan Schalm provided valuable research assistance in the first stage of this project. The author also learned much from his graduate students in healthy policy courses at the University of Regina and Queen's University in Kingston in which an earlier version of this profile was given a test run. Sections of this profile were also critiqued through public presentations at the University of Ottawa and Simon Fraser University.

The current series of Health System in Transition profiles has been prepared by the research directors and staff of the European Observatory on Health Systems and Policies. The European Observatory on Health Systems and Policies is a partnership between the WHO Regional Office for Europe, the governments of Belgium, Finland, Greece, Norway, Spain and Sweden, the Veneto Region of Italy, the European Investment Bank, the Open Society Institute, the World Bank, CRP-Santé Luxembourg, the London School of Economics and Political Science and the London School of Hygiene & Tropical Medicine.

The Observatory team working on the Health System in Transition profiles is led by Josep Figueras, Head of the Secretariat, and research directors Martin McKee, Elias Mossialos and Richard Saltman. Technical coordination is led by Susanne Grosse-Tebbe.

Giovanna Ceroni managed the production and copy-editing, with help from Nicole Satterly and with the support of Shirley and Johannes Frederiksen (layout). Administrative support for preparing the Health System profile on Canada was undertaken by Anna Maresso.

Special thanks are extended to the OECD for the data on health services. Thanks are also due to national statistical offices that have provided data.

This report reflects data available in May 2005.

Executive summary

T his Health System profile of Canada conforms to the pattern of similar country studies by the European Observatory on Health Systems and Policies to ensure some degree of comparability across systems. However, Canada is not a member of the European Union and not part of the WHO Regional Office for Europe's database. As a consequence, some comparisons draw upon the Organisation for Economic Co-operation and Development's health database in order to make comparisons (OECD 2004a).

Using the OECD database, five countries, including three European Union countries, are quantitatively compared to Canada. Australia, France, Sweden, the United Kingdom and the United States have been selected on the basis of political and health policy considerations as well as history, size and wealth.

Australia was selected because of the important similarities in government and the interesting comparisons in terms of the federal division of public health care responsibilities between the commonwealth and state governments. In addition to sharing one of Canada's two official languages, a systematic comparison with France is interesting because of its high public health care costs and quality. Sweden has often been used as a point of comparison because of its recent reform experience as well as recent public–private funding shifts. The United Kingdom was selected because the National Health Service was the model most understood by Canadian reformers in the formative stages of Medicare in Canada. For reasons of geographical, social and cultural proximity, the United States is an obvious point of comparison. In addition, however, the United States provides both a point of departure in terms of Medicare and Medicaid relative to Canadian Medicare, and a point of convergence in terms of the mixed and private portions of the Canadian system.

In the first section, this study provides the geographical, economic, and political context in which the Canadian health system is situated. This is followed by a brief survey of the health status of Canadians.

The second section lays out the organizational structure of Canadian health care. It begins with a concise history of the evolution of public health care followed by a contemporary overview of public, private and mixed health systems in the country. In terms of the public system, the governance and managerial systems are analysed in terms of their degree of decentralization or centralization. Issues of coverage, access, entitlements and benefits are also examined as well as emerging issues of quality improvement, choice, patient rights, patient safety, and citizen expectations and empowerment.

The third section examines the financial resources supporting Canadian health care. These include the sources of finance for public and private health care goods and services, the actual funding mechanisms, and the allocation of funding. Finally, the level and growth of health expenditures over the recent past is examined.

The fourth section deals with the planning, regulation and management of the Canadian health system. Since the provincial governments have primary jurisdiction over the organization and delivery of health and health care services, regulation and broad policy planning is provincial. There are, however, important exceptions to this, including the federal government's regulation of patented drugs and its extensive responsibilities for food and drug safety.

The fifth section reviews the non-financial inputs into the health system, in particular the physical and human resource infrastructure essential to health care delivery. In addition to surveying brick and mortar capital infrastructure, a section is devoted to the rapidly developing communications and information technology systems in Canadian health institutions and the state of medical equipment, devices and aids including the stock of advanced diagnostic equipment. Health care personnel groupings including doctors, nurses, dentists, pharmacists and many others are discussed in terms of their training and evolving functions. Trends concerning the number of health care personnel are also examined.

The sixth section describes the provision of health services, including the organization and delivery of services in various sectors as well as patient flows. These service sectors include: public health; primary care and ambulatory (outpatient) care; hospital and other specialized secondary care; prescription drug therapy; rehabilitation; long-term (institutional) care, home care and other community care; support services for informal caregivers; palliative care; mental health; dental health; alternative or complementary medicine; maternal and child health care; and health care targeting specific populations such as First Nations people and Inuit.

In the seventh section, the context and results of recent health care studies and reforms are summarized. The implementation of major reforms by both orders of government is described and analysed. This is accompanied by a preliminary prognosis concerning the future of health care in Canada, particularly public health care.

In the eighth section, an overall judgement of Canadian health care is made by assessing the extent to which the public (Medicare and public health), mixed (including prescription drugs, home, community and long-term care) and private systems (including most dental care and vision care): (1) distribute costs and benefits equitably; (2) allocate resources according to needs and preferences; (3) allocate sufficient resources efficiently; (4) are technically efficient; (5) are accountable; (6) empower patients and citizens; and (7) improve health.

The concluding section summarizes the current challenges and highlights areas that should be addressed in the next decade.

1. Introduction

1.1   Overview of the health system

Canada has a predominantly publicly financed health system with delivery effected through private (for-profit and not-for-profit) and public (arm's-length and direct) conduits. Beyond the 13 single-payer, universal systems of hospital and primary physician care defined as "insured services" under the federal Canada Health Act, the 13 provinces and territories vary considerably in terms of the financing, administration, delivery modes and range of public health care services. In addition to providing a health data, research and regulatory infrastructure, the federal government directly finances and administers a number of health services including those for First Nations people living on reserves, Inuit, members of the armed forces and the Royal Canadian Mounted Police, veterans, and inmates of federal penitentiaries.

As Fig. 1.1 illustrates, approximately 70% of total health expenditures occur in the public sector, largely through provincial governments which are primarily responsible for the administration of public health care in Canada. In most provinces and one territory, these services – hospital care, nursing homes and some home care and community care – are administered by geographically based regional health authorities.[1] All provincial governments remain responsible for administering prescription drug plans and paying physicians for their public health care services. The remaining 30% of health expenditures are in the private sector, paid either out-of-pocket or through private health insurance. This sector includes most dental and vision care services, some prescription drug care as well as virtually all complementary and alternative medicines and therapies. In addition, Canadians pay privately for some home care, community care and long-term care services and facilities.

---

[1] The exceptions are the province of Prince Edward Island and the territories of Yukon and Nunavut.

1.2   Geography and sociodemography

Canada is the second largest country in the world, with a land area of
9 093 507 km² (or 9 984 670 km² including inland water). The mainland spans
a distance of 5514 km from east to west, and 4634 km from north to south.
The country is bounded by the United States to the south and far north-west,
a country with almost ten times the population that exerts great cultural and
economic influence on the daily life of Canadians. The ten provinces (and their
respective capital cities) that make up Canada's federal system of government
are listed in order from west to east, followed by the northern territories from
west to east, in Table 1.1.

Fig. 1.1   Overview chart of health system

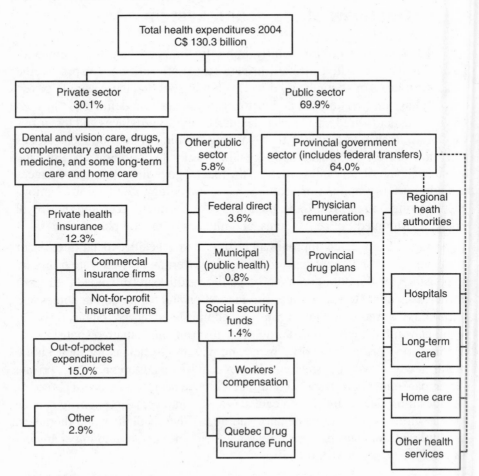

Source: CIHI 2004a.

Notes: Total health expenditures are forecast. Percentages may not add up due to rounding. National health expenditures are reported based on the principle of "responsibility for payment" rather than on the source of the funds. It is for this reason that federal health transfers to the provinces are included in the provincial government sector.

Private sector – the distribution of expenditures between private insurance, out-of-pocket and non-consumption is based on figures from 2002. No data was available for the distribution of expenditures between commercial and non-commercial insurance firms. "Other" includes non-patient revenues received by health care institutions such as donations and investment income; private spending on health-related capital construction and equipment; and health research funded by private sources.

Social security funds – not shown are the percentage values of workers' compensation boards (WCBs) and the Quebec Drug Insurance Fund. Worker compensation accounted for approximately C$1.2 billion or 1% of total health expenditures, while the Quebec drug plan accounted for the roughly C$0.5 billion remaining. Social security funds are social insurance programmes that are imposed and controlled by a government authority. They generally involve compulsory contributions by employees, employers or both, and the government authority determines the terms on which benefits are paid to recipients. Social security funds are distinguished from other social insurance programmes, the terms of which are determined by mutual agreement between individual employers and their employees. In Canada, social security funds include the health care spending by WCBs and the drug insurance fund component of the Quebec Ministry of Health and Social Services drug subsidy programme. Health spending by WCBs includes what the provincial boards commonly refer to as medical aid. Non-health related items often reported by the WCBs as medical aid expenditure such as funeral expenses, travel, clothing, etc., are removed.

The terrain of the country varies considerably from extensive mountain ranges in western Canada to the Great Lakes and the prairies of the south-western interior, and from the northern boreal shield to the vast tundra of the Arctic. The climate is northern in nature with a long and cold winter season experienced in almost all parts of the country.

Canada's population is almost 32 million. The census metropolitan area (CMA) of Toronto with 5.2 million inhabitants is the largest city, and Montreal with 3.4 million inhabitants is the second largest city. Located in between Toronto and Montreal, Ottawa is the capital of Canada. On average the country has 3.33 persons per km^2, but most of the population is concentrated in the country's more southern urban centres. A relatively small number of Canadians live in the immense rural and northern regions of the country. Most new immigrants live in Canada's largest cities, while the majority of Canada's Aboriginal peoples live on rural reserves, the poorer neighbourhoods of mid-sized or smaller prairie cities, and the northern regions of Canada, where they form the majority of the population in concentrated geographic areas.

At least four factors must be considered in terms of Canada's population health and health care delivery: demographic ageing, rural and remote populations, cultural diversity resulting from high rates of immigration, and Aboriginal health. Each of these issues is briefly summarized below.

Fig. 1.2   Map of Canada

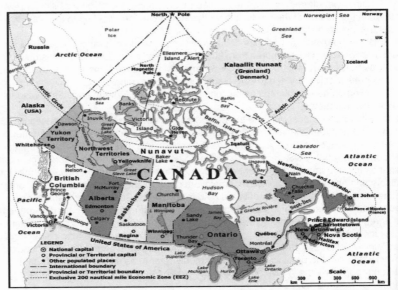

Source: Original map provided by The Atlas of Canada (http://atlas.gc.ca/) © 2005. Produced under licence from Her Majesty the Queen in Right of Canada, with permission of Natural Resources Canada.

Despite the demographic ageing of its population since 1970, Canada is still a young country with fewer older people than most European Union countries and Japan. Canada's age dependency ratio – defined as the ratio of children (1–14 years) plus the elderly (65 years and older) to the working-age population – is lower than the five comparator countries – Australia, France, Sweden, the United Kingdom and the United States – that have been selected on the basis of their useful comparability to Canada in terms of size and wealth as well as their respective political and health policy histories (Fig. 1.3).

Individuals aged 65 years and older made up 12.8% of the population in 2003 compared to 7.9% in 1970, but they are projected to constitute 20% of the population by 2025 (Canada 2002). The decrease in family size over time has served to cushion the age dependency ratio, with the total fertility rate declining from 2.3 children per woman in 1970 to approximately 1.5 in 2002, and the birth rate declining from 17.5 per 1000 population to 10.7 per 1000 over the same period (Table 1.2).

Using a definition of "rural" first developed by the OECD (1994), 30.4% of Canada's population lived in predominantly rural regions in 2001. Moreover, the three northern territories along with Saskatchewan, New Brunswick, Prince Edward Island, Nova Scotia and Newfoundland and Labrador have more than half of their respective populations living in predominantly rural

Table 1.1   Population in thousands, of provinces, and territories in 2004 (capital cities in parentheses)

Canada (Ottawa)	31 946
British Columbia (Victoria)	4 196
Alberta (Edmonton)	3 202
Saskatchewan (Regina)	995
Manitoba (Winnipeg)	1 170
Ontario (Toronto)	12 393
Quebec (Quebec City)	7 543
New Brunswick (Fredericton)	751
Nova Scotia (Halifax)	937
Prince Edward Island (Charlottetown)	138
Newfoundland and Labrador (St. John's)	517
Yukon (Whitehorse)	31
Northwest Territories (Yellowknife)	43
Nunavut (Iqaluit)	30

Source: Statistics Canada: CANSIM, Table 051–0001.

Notes: The population statistics are based on post-census data as of 1 July 2004.

Table 1.2   Population and demographic indicators

	1970	1980	1990	2000	2001	2002	2003
Total population (millions of persons)	21.3	24.5	27.7	30.7	31.0	31.4	31.6
Female population (% of total)	49.9	50.2	50.4	50.5	50.5	50.5	50.5
Age dependency ratio	59.5	47.4	47.0	46.5	46.0	45.6	45.2
Population 0–14 yrs (% of total)	30.1	22.7	20.7	19.2	18.9	18.6	18.3
Population 65 and over (% of total)	7.9	9.4	11.3	12.6	12.6	12.7	12.8
Birth rate (crude/per 1 000 people)	17.5	15.1	14.6	10.7	10.5	10.7	10.5
Death rate (crude/per 1 000 people)	7.3	7.0	6.9	7.1	7.1	7.1	7.2
Fertility rate (births per woman 15–49)	2.33	1.68	1.71	1.49	1.51	1.50	–
Population growth (annual %)	1.4	1.3	1.5	0.9	1.1	1.1	0.9

Sources: Statistics Canada: CANSIM, Tables 051–0001, 051–004; *The Daily*, 11 August 2003; *The Daily*, 9 April 2004.

Notes: Population statistics after 2001 are post-census estimates. The age dependency ratio is the ratio of the combined child population (aged 0 to 14) and elderly population (aged 65 and over) to the working age population (aged 15 to 64). This ratio is presented as the number of dependants for every 100 people in the working age population.

Figure 1.3   Age dependency ratio for Canada and selected countries, 2001

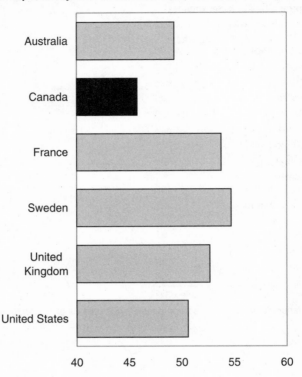

Source: OECD 2004a.

regions (Agriculture and Agri-Food Canada 2002). Those segments of rural populations that are far from metropolitan centres – defined as "rural non-metro-adjacent regions" and "rural northern and remote regions" – present enormous challenges to the delivery of health care in terms of the range, quality and cost of services offered. Canadians in these regions suffer lower health status while having greater difficulty accessing even basic primary care services, much less specialized health care services (Canada 2002).

High post-Second World War immigration to Canada has created a culturally diverse population. Based on the 2001 census, 18.4% of Canadian residents were born outside of the country, a majority of whom came from non-English-speaking countries. In terms of the population as a whole, 33.6% of the population are originally of British origin, 15.9% of French origin, 29.5% of other European origin, 9.9% of Asian origin, 4.4% of Aboriginal origin, and the remaining of Latin American, African, Caribbean and Arab origin (Statistics Canada 2001a). Most recent immigrants come from outside of Europe and do not have English or French as their first language. They are clustered in Canada's largest cities putting pressure on health care facilities in those areas to provide services in ways that can overcome cultural and linguistic barriers to access.

Canadians that reported some Aboriginal ancestry made up 4.4% of the total population in 2001. Of these 1.3 million, 74% identified themselves as North American Indian, Metis or Inuit, while the remaining 26% were of undefined Aboriginal identity. Almost 50% of Aboriginal Canadians are status First Nations people living on and off reservations. A further 26% are non-status Indians, many of whom are concentrated in urban areas, 22% are Metis living mainly in western Canada, and 3.4% are Inuit who live in the Arctic regions of Canada (Statistics Canada 2001a).

Aboriginal peoples suffer disproportionately from chronic diseases and conditions such as diabetes, hypertension, heart disease, tuberculosis, HIV and fetal alcohol syndrome. In addition, the death rate due to injuries and poisoning is considerably higher for First Nations people and Inuit than for the total Canadian population (Senate 2001b). Indeed, First Nations people living on reserves suffer from physical injuries at a rate four times that of all Canadians (CIHI 2004a). As a result, Aboriginal Canadians account for higher use (and higher cost) of health care services than other Canadians.

For constitutional and historical reasons, the funding, administration and delivery of Aboriginal health services are highly complex and fragmented. In addition, few of these services are delivered in a manner that respects Aboriginal culture, language and traditional healing services (Lavoie 2004; Canada 2002). However, the broader social determinants of health, including relative poverty and marginalization, largely explain the poorer health outcomes of Aboriginal Canadians relative to other Canadians, and consequent greater use of public health care services.

1.3   Economic context

Canada is an advanced industrial economy with a substantial resource base. Living standards are among the highest in the world and GDP per capita (measured as purchasing-power-parity adjusted US dollars) was US $27 130 in 2001. Between 1998 and 2003, the very period that Canadian health care costs were growing rapidly, Canadian GDP per capita grew more rapidly than any other G7 country including the United States. Since that time, Canadian economic growth has slowed slightly as a consequence of a number of factors including the dampening of exports due to the rising Canadian dollar as well as outbreaks of Severe Acute Respiratory Syndrome (SARS) and Bovine Spongiform Encephalopathy (BSE, or "mad cow" disease) in 2003.

1.4   Political context

Canada is a constitutional monarchy based upon a Westminster-style parliamentary democracy. It is also a federation with two constitutionally recognized orders of government. The first order is the central or "federal" government, generally a reference to the democratically elected members of parliament (MPs) of the House of Commons, although formally it also includes the appointed members of an upper house known as the Senate of Canada. Senators are appointed on a regional basis by the Prime Minister of Canada.

Although the provinces (and territories) are primarily responsible for health care in Canada, the federal government has jurisdiction over prescription drug regulation and safety, as well as for the financing and administration of a range of health benefits and services for First Nations and Inuit people that are not included in provincial and territorial insured health care programmes, as well as health care services for members of the Canadian armed forces and the Royal Canadian Mounted Police, veterans and inmates in federal penitentiaries. In addition, the federal government also has important responsibilities in the domains of public health, health research and health data collection. Through its use of spending power in the form of fiscal transfers to the provinces and territories, the federal government upholds and enforces the national dimensions of insured hospitals and physicians as defined under the Canada Health Act.

The provinces constitute the second order of government. Provincial governments have become increasingly important in the lives of Canadians because the provinces bear the principal responsibility for social policy, including health and education as well as social assistance and social services. While responsible for the administration of public health care, the provinces deliver very few health services directly. Most public health services are organized or delivered by regional health authorities that have been delegated the responsibility to administer services within defined geographic areas. Most physicians work in their own private clinics but receive remuneration based upon fee-for-service schedules that are periodically renegotiated with provincial governments.

As measured by relative revenues and expenditures, Canada has become an increasingly decentralized federation since the early 1960s (Marchildon

Table 1.3   Macroeconomic indicators, 1990, 1996 and 2000–2003

	1990	1996	2000	2001	2002	2003
GDP (billions current C$)	679.9	836.9	1 075.6	1 107.5	1 154.9	1 214.6
GDP per capita (current C$)	24 548	28 262	35 047	35 700	36 826	38 400
Real GDP (billions 1997 C$)	757.2	859.1	1 033.3	1 047.6	1 083.9	1 101.6
GDP, PPP (billions US$)	515.4	676.4	873.4	911.2	951.9	–
GDP per capita, PPP (US$)	18 604	23 338	28 107	28 811	30 300	–
Real annual GDP growth rate (%)	-1.2	2.7	4.2	1.4	3.5	1.6
Inflation rate (GDP deflator per year)	3.3	1.6	3.8	1.0	0.9	3.4
Inflation rate (CPI % per year)	4.8	1.6	2.7	2.6	2.2	3.5
CPI (1992 = 100)	93.3	105.9	113.5	116.4	119.0	123.2
Labour force (millions)	14.2	14.9	16.0	16.3	16. 7	17.1
Unemployment rate (% population)	8.1	9.6	6.8	7.2	7.7	7.5
Real interest rate (prime rate %)	7.8	2.6	4.3	3.3	0.6	2.5
Exchange rate (US$ per Canadian $)	0.86	0.73	0.67	0.65	0.64	0.71
Low income cut-off (% population)	15.1	18.5	14.6	13.3	13.7	–
General government financial balance (% GDP)	-5.9	-2.8	3.1	1.8	1.3	–
Current account balance (billions of C$ – seasonally adjusted)	-5.7	0.3	9.0	2.8	4.9	6.7
Value added in all goods producing industries (% real GDP by industry)	32.4	32.3	33.0	31.1	31.3	31.5
in agriculture	3.0	2.7	2.3	2.1	2.1	2.3
in industrial production	23.0	24.3	25.6	23.6	23.9	23.8
Value added in service producing industries (% real GDP by industry)	67.2	67.5	67.1	69.3	68.8	68.8

Sources: Finance Canada 2003; OECD 2004b; Statistics Canada: CANSIM, 2004; and *The Daily*, 26 February 2004.

Notes: Real GDP figures are expenditure-based, seasonally adjusted, chained 1997 dollars. Annual figures are based on fourth quarter results. Current account balance is as of fourth quarter. Low income cut-off (LICO) is used to distinguish "low income" family units from "other" family units. A family unit is considered "low income" when the proportion of its income devoted to food, shelter and clothing is below the cut-off for its family size and its community. Statistics Canada is currently using LICOs based on 1992 family spending data, updated to allow for inflation as reflected in the consumer price index (CPI).

1995). This trend has, in part, been driven by the struggle of successive Quebec governments for greater autonomy from the federal government. Following suit, other provinces have also sought greater autonomy. In recent years, the provinces have consistently demanded greater fiscal resources from the federal government to meet their growing public health care expenditures while also demanding less federal conditionality and greater flexibility, in terms of how they spend those same federal health transfers.

Municipalities are not recognized in the constitution of Canada as autonomous orders of government. Instead, they are treated as "creatures of the provinces". Municipal governments, including county governments in some provinces, are delegated authority and responsibility by the provinces (and territories) for the delivery of local public services and infrastructure. Historically, municipalities played a role, albeit modest, in the administration and delivery of health services, but the Saskatchewan model of single-payer Medicare, with a payment system centralized in provincial governments, was eventually adopted by other provinces and territories (Taylor 1987).

Canada also has three northern territories. While the territories are creatures of the federal government in constitutional terms, they have been delegated ever more extensive authorities and responsibilities. In practice, the three territories behave like provinces and are gradually moving towards full provincial status. Moreover, they have followed the provincial pattern in terms of organizing and administering their own territorial public health care systems.

Elections take place on average every four years for the federal House of Commons as well as provincial and territorial legislatures under a "first-past-the-post"[2] electoral system based on federal, provincial and territorial constituencies and largely within the context of competitive and adversarial political parties.[3] Political parties are also "federalized", with provincial political parties of a particular stripe enjoying considerable autonomy from federal parties of the same political family.

The Prime Minister is the leader of the majority party in the House of Commons and appoints the cabinet of ministers. In December 2003, Paul Martin of the Liberal Party of Canada became Prime Minister. He succeeded Jean Chrétien, who had been Prime Minister since 1993. Recently, both prime ministers, along with provincial and territorial first ministers, have been instrumental in negotiating public health care priorities through three major intergovernmental accords (CICS 2000, 2003, 2004).

---

[2] Each voter selects one candidate. All votes are counted and the candidate with the most votes in a defined geographic constituency is the winner.

[3] With majority Aboriginal populations, the territorial governments of Nunavut and the Northwest Territories have eschewed adversarial party-dominated government in favour of consensual (non-party) government.

Canada is a founding member of the United Nations and, because of its history as a self-governing colony within the British Empire, is a member of the Commonwealth of Nations. Because of its status as a French- as well as English-speaking jurisdiction, Canada is also a member of the Organisation Internationale de la Francophonie, as are the provinces of Quebec and New Brunswick.

Global health forms part of Canadian foreign policy and Canada is a signatory to several international treaties that recognize the right to health, the most important of which are the Universal Declaration of Human Rights (1948) and the International Covenant on Economic, Social and Cultural Rights (1976). In 1991, Canada ratified the United Nation Convention on the Rights of the Child and its provisions concerning the health and health care rights of children. In 1997, Canada became a member of the World Intellectual Property Organization (WIPO) Copyright Treaty, which has important implications for prescription drug patenting as well as research and development in the medical sector generally.[4]

Canada is an active participant in the World Health Organization (WHO) and its Regional Office, the Pan American Health Organization (PAHO). Under the auspices of WHO, the Framework Convention on Tobacco Control (2003) attempts to "strengthen and broaden public health measures to reduce smoking" and thereby reduce its deleterious health consequences throughout the world. As a country that has succeeded in reducing its smoking rate dramatically over the past few decades, Canada was a leader in the negotiation of this landmark convention and in initiating a more global effort to reduce tobacco consumption (Kapur 2003).

In addition, Canada has been acting as secretariat to the global health security initiative involving 180 countries since 2001. The secretariat's tasks include preparing and disseminating a vaccine procurement protocol and developing coursework in containment and isolation for smallpox and other contagious diseases. Canada has also taken a lead role with WHO in identifying chronic disease prevention and control, helping establish a Framework Agreement for Cooperation on Chronic Diseases in 2005.

Canada is also a member of the World Trade Organization (WTO) and, with the United States and Mexico, is a member of the North American Free Trade Agreement (NAFTA). NAFTA and the General Agreement on Trade in Services (GATS) under the WTO are very broad in their scope but both contain provisions that ostensibly protect public health care services from coming under these trade rules. NAFTA, for example, exempts all "social services established

---

[4] WIPO is one of 16 specialized agencies of the United Nations.

or maintained for a public purpose" from its trade and investment liberalization provisions. On the other hand, GATS only applies to those services or sectors that are explicitly made subject to the agreement, and countries such as Canada have chosen not to include its own public health care services in GATS (Canada 2002; Ouellet 2004).

None the less, some Canadians remain anxious about future health care services coming under the purview of international trade laws. This anxiety is fuelled by the fact that, in addition to the large private sector of health services in Canada, there are also private elements in the administration, funding and delivery of health care, and private interests in other countries may eventually demand "national treatment" in order to compete on an equal playing field with these domestic interests (Epps and Flood 2002; Johnson 2004b). There are also other concerns. One relates to the one-way ratchet effect of privatization. If the Canadian Government chose to move public health services into the private sector, the WTO rules do not permit the national government to "re-protect" these services at a later date. A second concern involves NAFTA's rules which require compensation to be paid to foreign firms for loss of profit opportunities as a consequence of regulatory change (Sanger and Sinclair 2004; Grishaber-Otto and Sinclair 2004).

1.5   Health status

With some important exceptions, Canadians enjoy good health relative to other countries. Table 1.4 illustrates the improvements in the standard and quality of life of Canadians since 1970, including life expectancy at birth, one of the most common summary measures of health status. Of the many factors that have contributed to this improvement, three stand out: increases in wealth and its more equitable distribution; improvements in "lifestyle" factors including disease prevention and public health measures; and the quality of, and access to health care. Since the late 1960s, life expectancy at birth has risen roughly 1 year for every 5 calendar years. By the end of the 20th century, Canada ranked 5th among all OECD countries.

Potential years of life lost (PYLL), as defined and measured by Statistics Canada, is the number of years lost "prematurely" by deaths prior to age 75. In 1960, PYLL was 9395 years lost per 100 000 people. By 2000, PYLL had dropped to 3571 (Table 1.4), a significant improvement and one that places Canada seventh among all countries in the OECD (see Table 8.2).

Since its *World health report 2000*, the World Health Organization has been encouraging its member states to collect data on disability-adjusted life expectancy (DALE) in order to compare the extent to which societies are not only lengthening people's lives but also improving the quality of their lives by assessing the number of years that people live without disabling conditions (WHO 2000). In addition to the safety and quality of the environment in which people live and work, DALE also measures the effectiveness of health promotion and injury and illness prevention programming. Based upon the work done

Table 1.4   Life expectancy and mortality indicators (per 100 000 population^a), 1970–2001

	1970	1980	1990	1995	2000	2001
Life expectancy at birth, females	–	78.9	80.8	81.1	82.0	82.2
Life expectancy at birth, males	–	71.7	74.4	75.1	76.7	77.1
Life expectancy at birth, total population at birth	–	75.3	77.6	78.2	79.4	79.7
Infant mortality (deaths/1 000 live births)	18.8	10.4	6.8	6.0	5.3	5.2
Maternal mortality (deaths/100 000 live births)	20.0	8.0	2.5	4.5	3.4	7.8
Potential years of lost life (per 100 000, age 0–74)	–	6 250	4 716	4 180	3 571	–
All malignant neoplasms (mortality)	183.4	185.8	191.7	180.7	175.7	–
Lung cancer	30.5	42.9	51.1	48.5	46.9	–
Prostate cancer	24.0	25.7	30.1	31.0	24.6	–
Breast cancer	30.2	29.7	31.3	28.7	24.5	–
Colorectal cancer	30.9	25.0	21.1	20.0	17.1	–
Digestive diseases (mortality)	31.8	32.5	24.7	22.6	21.3	–
All circulatory disease (mortality)	488.4	379.1	260.7	227.3	191.5	–
Acute myocardial infarction	–	139.9	86.1	66.5	52.1	–
Cerebrovascular disease	100.8	70.2	47.6	43.4	37.8	–
Ischaemic heart diseases	309.4	231.8	154.2	128.8	108.5	–
Respiratory disease (mortality)	64.7	52.3	55.9	53.6	44.3	–
Pneumonia and influenza	36.1	22.3	22.0	19.7	–	–
Infectious and parasitic disease deaths (mortality)	7.0	3.6	7.8	10.2	8.3	–
HIV	–	–	3.2	5.0	1.4	–
Mental and behavioural disorders (mortality)	2.7	6.1	9.6	13.5	13.6	–
External causes (mortality)	70.9	65.5	46.9	42.4	38.2	–

Sources: OECD 2004a; Statistics Canada 2003 and CANSIM.
^{a} Unless otherwise stated

by Mathers et al. (2000), Canada was ranked 9th out of 191 countries on the DALE indicator.

Infant mortality rates are, for the most part, a reflection of the various determinants of health, including education, housing, nutrition and standards of living, but they can also demonstrate the impact of primary health care initiatives and, in particular, the quality of prenatal care (Canada 2002). Although the infant mortality rate has declined steadily since 1970 (see Table 1.4), it is important to note that Canada only ranks 17th among OECD countries.[5] In contrast, Canada ranks 11th among OECD countries in perinatal mortality, defined as the number of deaths that occur between the 28th week of pregnancy and the first month of the baby's life (OECD 2004a). It should be noted that the perinatal mortality rate is a better indicator of the quality of (and access to) health care than the infant mortality rate, which is more sensitive to general social conditions (see Table 8.2).

Table 1.4 also sets out the main causes of death in Canada from cancer to circulatory, respiratory, digestive and infectious diseases. To the extent that death and survival rates provide a measure of the timeliness of response of the health system to specific health problems, except in the case of cerebrovascular diseases where Canada ranks in the top two OECD countries (see Table 8.3), the picture that emerges for other diseases is decidedly mixed, a picture that is reinforced in a comparative study of five countries including Canada recently conducted by the Commonwealth Fund's International Working Group on Quality Indicators (Hussey et al. 2004).

In the case of all cancers, Canada has made limited progress since 1970 and is currently ranked 15th among OECD countries in terms of mortality (see Table 8.3). Similarly, Canada has fared average to poor in terms of progress on respiratory and infectious disease. More progress has been made in reducing deaths from digestive diseases and Canada now has a ranking of 9th among OECD countries. Canada's best performance to date has been on addressing circulatory disease with the death rate almost halved within three decades (see Table 1.4), with the country ranking 5th in the OECD for all circulatory system diseases (OECD 2004a).

In all these cases, however, factors other than the health care system may be more important in determining outcomes. The DALE indicator, in particular, has been criticized for methodological shortcomings specific to its construction. In addition, DALE and other aggregate measures inevitably combine the effects of health care with those that are a product of the broader social environment.

---

[5] It should be noted, however, that in Canada, the United States and the Nordic countries, very premature babies are registered as live births thereby increasing these countries' mortality rates relative to other countries.

Recently, the Canadian Institute for Health Information (CIHI) has put considerable effort into constructing indicators that provide an accurate index of the performance of the health care system (Table 1.5). Ambulatory care sensitive conditions – such as pneumonia, asthma, hypertension, angina, diabetes and epileptic convulsions – are a measure of access to appropriate medical care, particularly primary medical care. While not all admissions for ambulatory care sensitive conditions are avoidable, it is assumed that appropriate prior ambulatory care could prevent the onset of this type of illness or condition, or control an acute episodic illness or condition, or manage a chronic disease or condition. In the four years since 2000, the admission rate for ambulatory care sensitive conditions has fallen quite consistently.

Table 1.5   Selected CIHI health system performance indicators, 2000–2004 (age-standardized hospitalization rates per 100 000 population)

	2000	2001	2002	2003	2004
Ambulatory care sensitive conditions	447	411	401	370	346
Pneumonia and influenza	1 241	1 273	1 297	1 092	–
Hip fractures	618	599	575	575	554

Source: CIHI discharge abstract and hospital morbidity databases.

Similarly, high rates of hospital admission for pneumonia and influenza can be prevented through accessible influenza and pneumococcal immunization programmes, health education and effective primary care. The results in Table 1.5 are ambiguous and the lower hospitalization rate in 2003 may simply reflect a less severe outbreak of influenza that year.

While hip fractures among older people can occur for a number of reasons, some hospitalizations can be avoided through improving the quality of care in, as well as the safety of, long-term care (nursing home) facilities. Some hip fracture hospitalizations can also be prevented through more careful prescription of psychotropic medications or by offering non-drug therapies and advice including physiotherapy, occupational therapy and rehabilitation services. On this measure, there has been some decrease since 2000 but more time is needed to determine whether there will be a sustainable improvement in long-term care and medication management (Table 1.5).

While Table 1.5 shows a general improvement for at least two indicators, a long-time series combined with a large basket of indicators will be required for a more definitive assessment of the performance of the Canadian health system.

In the spring and summer of 2003, Canada was rocked by the outbreak of an infectious and deadly viral illness known as severe acute respiratory syndrome (SARS). By August 2003, there were over 400 probable and suspect SARS cases in Canada as well as 44 deaths in the Greater Toronto Area. More than 100 health care workers became ill and three ultimately died of SARS. As the hardest-hit country outside of Asia, Canada in general, and Toronto in particular, became the focus of public and international attention, with WHO issuing travel advice recommending against non-essential travel to Toronto from 2 to 29 April 2003 (Health Canada 2003a).

As a consequence of the SARS outbreak in Toronto, and the difficulties associated with the public health response by the City of Toronto and the governments of Ontario and Canada, Health Canada established a National Advisory Committee on SARS and Public Health chaired by Dr David Naylor of the University of Toronto. The committee's mandate was to report on the crisis and then recommend improvements to Canada's public infrastructure and collaboration among governments to deal with public health emergencies, as well as to make some directional recommendations on the future of public health in Canada. Towards the end of 2003, the committee delivered its report, and using in part the example of the Centers for Disease Control and Prevention (CDC) in the United States, recommended the establishment of a similar public health organization in Canada (Health Canada 2003a). In 2004, the Public Health Agency of Canada was established along with the country's Chief Public Health Officer.

Table 1.6 sets out some of the more common lifestyle factors influencing health status in Canada. It is noteworthy that alcohol and tobacco consumption have dropped considerably relative to consumption levels in the 1980s. Nevertheless, it is estimated that approximately 45 000 Canadians die each year from smoking-related illnesses (Makomaski-Illing and Kaiserman 1999) that in turn involve C$2.4 billion worth of health care expenditures (Stephens et al. 2000). In addition, it appears that alcohol consumption has begun to creep up since 1996, perhaps a reflection of what economist and demographer David Foot (2001) has described as the echo of the post-war baby boom.

Unfortunately, more Canadians are obese today than in the past creating a myriad of health problems for the individuals affected and growing demands on the health system in general (Katzmarzyk 2002). In 2003 approximately 7.9 million adults aged 18 and older were overweight (body mass index (BMI) 25–29.9) and roughly 3.5 million were obese (BMI ≥30) based upon a measure of body mass (BMI) that is calculated on weight divided by height squared. This means that roughly 25% of the Canadian population is overweight while approximately 11% is obese. Moreover, obesity is becoming more prevalent among Canadian children, a situation with dire implications for the longer-term

Table 1.6   Factors influencing health status, 1981–2002

	1981	1986	1991	1996	1997	1998	1999	2000	2001	2002
Alcohol consumption (litres per capita, 15+)	97.8	92.2	83.4	77.8	78.5	79.8	80.8	81.2	80.6	81.1
Daily smokers (% of population)	32.8	28.3	25.9	24.5	23.8	23.7	20.9	19.8	18.0	–
Total calories intake (per capita)	2 337	2 411	2 356	2 585	–	2 715	2 725	2 732	2 757	2 788
Obese population (% of total population BMI>30kg/m²)	–	–	12.2	12.2	14.6	–	14.5	–	14.9	–
Measles immunizations (% of children >2 years of age)	–	–	–	97.0	96.0	96.2	–	–	–	–
Diphtheria, pertussis and tetanus (DPT) immunizations (% of children >2 years of age)	–	–	–	87.1	86.8	84.2	–	–	–	–

Sources: OECD 2004a; Statistics Canada 2002 and CANSIM, Tables 104–0009, 104–0027.

Notes: Calorie intake is consumption per day/per person. Alcohol consumption is measured in litres per person by retail weight. Immunization rates are estimates only.

health of the population as this will increase the incidence of Type 2 diabetes, gallbladder disease, osteoarthritis and other obesity-related conditions (CIHI 2004a). Although lower than the United States and the United Kingdom, Canada's obesity rates are considerably higher than most continental European countries as well as Australia (OECD 2001).

Immunizations through public health programmes and effective primary care can prevent measles, diphtheria, tetanus and pertussis. The organization and delivery of both measles and diphtheria, pertussis and tetanus (DTP) immunization programmes varies considerably in Canada depending on the regional health authority or the provincial/territorial government in question. While measles immunization is relatively successful, such that Canada ranks 7th among OECD countries, DPT immunization of children is so poorly done that Canada ranks 19th (see Table 8.2). Partly in response to this situation, the Conference of Federal, Provincial and Territorial Deputy Ministers of Health began work on a national immunization strategy in 1999.

Aboriginal Canadians suffer disproportionately from diseases that can be prevented through immunization. They are also far more likely to suffer from high-risk factors that negatively influence health because of high consumption of tobacco and alcohol (CIHI 2004a). The poor health status of Canada's Aboriginal population has elicited much comment and concern in recent years, including a major study initiated by the Royal Commission on Aboriginal Peoples (Canada 1996). While the health outcomes of Aboriginal Canadians are a little closer to the Canadian average today than they were two or three decades ago, a deep disparity none the less persists. Many of the reasons are rooted in the social and economic structure of Canadian society and a historic degree of marginalization and prejudice that few immigrant groups to Canada have suffered (Lemchuk-Favel and Jock 2004).

2. Organizational structure

2.1 Historical background

The administration and delivery of public health care in Canada are highly decentralized. This defining characteristic has been shaped by at least three factors: provincial responsibility for the administration and delivery of most public health care services; the historic arm's-length relationship between government on the one hand and the hospital sector and physicians on the other; and recent regionalization reforms in which sub-provincial organizations are now responsible for the allocation of most health resources.

Historically, hospitals in Canada were encouraged by provincial government subsidies to admit and treat all patients, irrespective of their ability to pay. The government of Ontario set the template through its Charity Aid Act of 1874 in which not-for-profit municipal, charitable and religious denomination-based (mainly Catholic and Protestant) hospitals were obliged to accept patients on the basis of medical need in return for a per diem reimbursement and some regulatory oversight by provincial governments. Private-for-profit hospitals were excluded, thus limiting the already small number of such hospitals in Canada. At the same time, however, the proliferation of municipal and not-for-profit hospitals voluntarily serving a public purpose meant that there were few state-owned and controlled hospitals (Boychuk 1999). The major exceptions to this evolution were the provincially administered mental hospitals that emerged in the twentieth century in response to the poor state of private and nongovernmental asylums. Provincial institutions such as the cottage hospitals in the coastal fishing communities of Newfoundland and the inpatient institutions for the treatment of tuberculosis and cancer were also run directly by some governments.

Table 2.1   Chronology of the evolution of public health care, 1945–1984

1945	Federal offer of cost-sharing for public health insurance during Dominion-Provincial post-war reconstruction conference rejected by some provinces
1947	Saskatchewan implements universal hospital insurance
1948	Federal government introduces National Health Grants Program to strengthen public health initiatives and assist provinces in building hospital infrastructure
1949	British Columbia introduces a universal hospital services plan
1950	Alberta establishes user fee-based hospital insurance via municipalities
1957	Federal cost-sharing of provincial hospitalization provided in the Hospital Insurance and Diagnostic Services Act and implemented over next few years
1962	Saskatchewan introduction of universal medical (physician) care insurance accompanied by a bitter, province-wide, doctors' strike
1964	Royal Commission on Health Services, chaired by Emmett Hall, recommends national system of medical care insurance based mainly on the Saskatchewan model
1966	Medical Care Act passed in federal parliament
1968	Implementation of Medical Care Act through federal-provincial negotiation and federal transfers on cost-sharing basis
1972	Yukon is last jurisdiction to join the Medicare plan
1974	Lalonde report on the determinants of health is published
1977	Established Programs Financing Act (EPF) replaces federal cost-sharing with federal tax and cash transfers to provinces tied to growth in GNP and population
1980	Emmett Hall reports to federal Minister of Health and Welfare on impact of physician, hospital and health facility billing practices on accessibility to Medicare
1984	Canada Health Act passed: mandatory financial deductions from federal transfer to provinces for user fees and extra charges

As was the case for hospital care for the indigent, Ontario initially led the way in the provision of public medical care. In 1882, Ontario's Public Health Act established a broad range of public health measures, a permanent board of health and the country's first medical officer of health. In 1914, Ontario introduced workers' compensation legislation that provided medical, hospital and rehabilitation care for all entitled workers in the event of any work-related accident or injury in return for workers giving up their legal right to sue employers. This legislation, and the Workers' Compensation Board (WCB) that it established, became the model for the remaining provinces. Less than two decades later, Ontario would also be the first jurisdiction to establish a province-wide medical service plan for all social assistance recipients (Naylor 1986; Taylor 1987).

While most provinces followed Ontario's lead in terms of targeted public health and public health insurance, the provinces in western Canada laid the groundwork for universal hospital and medical care that would eventually become known as Medicare. In 1916, the Government of Saskatchewan amended its municipal legislation to facilitate the establishment of hospital districts as well as the employment of salaried doctors providing a range of health services, including public health, general medical and maternity as well as minor surgery. These hospitals and physicians served all residents of the participating municipalities on the same terms and conditions (Taylor 1987; Houston 2002).

During the 1920s, the Government of Alberta responded to the pressure for state health insurance by establishing a commission to examine a range of public health insurance possibilities. The report of the Legislative Commission on Medical and Hospital Services was delivered in 1929. While the report stated that state health insurance, administered either by the province or through the municipalities, was feasible, the Government of Alberta concluded that the cost to the public treasury was too high, and did not implement the recommendation.

In 1929, the Government of British Columbia appointed a Royal Commission on State Health Insurance and Medical Benefits. In a report delivered three years later, the commission recommended a social insurance health scheme, with compulsory contributions for all employees beneath a threshold level of income. The provincial government passed legislation in 1936 but the bill's implementation was postponed, and then ultimately abandoned, when the government failed to secure the cooperation of the provincial association of physicians.

As a result of the Great Depression of the 1930s, a growing number of Canadians were unable to pay for hospital or physician services. At the same time, government revenues fell so rapidly that it became more difficult for governments to consider underwriting the cost of health services. Despite this, Newfoundland introduced a state-operated cottage hospital and medical care programme to serve some of the isolated "outport" fishing communities in 1934, 15 years before it joined the Canadian federation. By the time Newfoundland (since renamed Newfoundland and Labrador) joined the Canadian confederation in 1949, 47% of the population of the province were covered under the cottage hospital programme (Taylor 1987).

The next major push for public health coverage came from the federal government as part of its wartime planning and post-war and reconstruction efforts. In the 1945/1946 Dominion-Provincial Reconstruction Conference, the federal government put forward a broad package of social security and fiscal changes, part of which included an offer to cost share 60% of public hospital and medical care insurance. This offer was ultimately rejected because of concerns, mainly held by Ontario and Quebec, about the administrative and tax arrangements that would have accompanied the comprehensive social security programme. The failure of this federal-provincial conference forced a more piecemeal approach to the introduction of public health care in the post-war years, with the western Canadian provinces in the forefront of these new initiatives.

In 1947, Saskatchewan implemented a universal hospital services plan popularly known as hospitalization. Unlike private insurance policies, no limitation was placed on the number of "entitlement days" as long as the hospital services rendered were medically necessary, and no distinction was made between basic services and optional extras. In addition to hospital services, coverage included X-rays, laboratory services and some prescription drugs. These design features did much to eliminate the possibility of a separate tier of private hospital insurance growing up alongside hospitalization. Saskatchewan would be financially aided by the introduction of national health grants by the federal government in 1948 (Johnson 2004a). The grants included money for provincial initiatives in public health, mental health, venereal disease, tuberculosis and general health surveys as well as hospital construction (Taylor 1987).

In 1949, the Government of British Columbia implemented a universal hospitalization scheme based upon the Saskatchewan model. One year later, the Government of Alberta introduced its own hospitalization scheme through subsidies paid to those municipalities that agreed to provide public hospital coverage to residents. Both programmes encountered challenges in their implementation. In the British Columbia case, a number of implementation problems led to a revamping of the programme after a new government was elected in 1952. In Alberta, the partial and voluntary nature of the initiative meant that on the eve of the introduction of national hospitalization in 1957, 25% of the population was still not benefiting from public hospital insurance.

In 1955, the Government of Ontario announced its willingness to implement public coverage for hospital and diagnostic services if the federal government would agree to share the cost with the province. One year later, the federal government agreed in principle to cost-sharing such services. In 1957, the federal Hospital Insurance and Diagnostic Services Act was passed in Parliament. This law set out the common conditions that provinces would have to satisfy in order to receive shared-cost financing through federal transfers. In 1958, the provinces of Saskatchewan, British Columbia, Alberta, Manitoba and Newfoundland agreed to work within the federal framework of hospitalization. One year later, Ontario, Nova Scotia, New Brunswick and Prince Edward Island signed on. Quebec did not agree until 1961, shortly after the election of a government dedicated to modernizing the provincial welfare state (Taylor 1987).

With the introduction of federal cost-sharing for hospitalization, the province of Saskatchewan was financially able to proceed with universal coverage for physician services. However, the introduction of the prepaid, public administered "Medicare" plan triggered a bitter, province-wide doctors' strike that lasted for 23 days in 1962. The strike officially ended with a compromise known as the Saskatoon Agreement in which the nature and mechanism of payment emphasized the contractual autonomy of physicians from the provincial government (Naylor 1986; Taylor 1987).

In 1964, the Royal Commission on Health Services, commonly known as the Hall Commission, delivered its report to the Prime Minister. The Hall Commission recommended that the federal government encourage provinces beyond Saskatchewan to introduce public coverage for physician care through cost-sharing (Canada 1964). In 1966, the federal government passed the Medical Care Act with federal cost-sharing transfers to begin flowing in 1968 to the provinces conforming to the four general principles of universality, public administration, comprehensiveness and portability. By 1972, all the provinces and territories had implemented universal public insurance for physician care.

Thus, it took a quarter century from the time that hospitalization was first introduced by a province until the time that public insurance for physicians was implemented by all jurisdictions, for the establishment of a universal public health care insurance system. This system, run as individual single-payer schemes by the provinces and territories but tied together nationally through a set of common principles set in federal law, is commonly known by Canadians as "Medicare" (Phillips and Swan 1996).

The 1970s marked a period of rapid expansion of public coverage and subsidies for health care services well beyond hospital and medical care by the provinces and territories. These included prescription drug plans as well as programmes, services and subsidies for home care and long-term (institution-based) care. Lacking any national principles or federal funding, however, these initiatives varied considerably across the country depending on the fiscal capacity and policy ambitions of the province or territory in question.

During this same period, the federal government initiated much new thinking concerning the basic determinants of health beyond medical care, including biological factors, lifestyle choices and environmental, social and economic conditions. In 1974, the Canadian Minister of Health, Marc Lalonde, released a report – *A new perspective on the health of Canadians* – summarizing this new approach (McKay 2001). The Lalonde report triggered further work in Canada and this work, with its emphasis on the "upstream" determinants of health, influenced subsequent provincial studies and provided the intellectual foundation for the "wellness" reforms introduced by the provinces by the early 1990s.

By 1977, the federal government and the provinces agreed to replace the cost-sharing transfer with a block transfer funding mechanism. The Established Programs Financing arrangement gave the provinces greater flexibility in terms of how they used federal transfers. No longer required to spend federal money on hospitals and medical care, provinces could now apply transfer money to health expenditures in general, including drug plans and home care. In return, the federal government was able to cap its growth in health transfer to the growth in the economy rather than be tied to a formula that required federal health transfers to match provincial health expenditures.

While the practices of physicians charging extra to patients and hospitals charging patients user fees predated Established Programs Financing, these practices seemed to accelerate afterwards. As a consequence, the federal Minister of Health ordered an external review. Emmett Hall was asked to undertake this "check-up on Medicare" and his 1980 report made a number of specific recommendations to deal with the user fees imposed by some hospitals or clinics and extra charges by some physicians, including amending federal law to state that such practices impeded reasonable access to health care and therefore were contrary to the intent and purpose of Medicare as originally designed (Hall 1980). A subsequent parliamentary committee agreed with Hall and suggested that federal transfers be withheld, on a graduated basis, where a provincial plan impeded reasonable access by permitting user fees or extra charges.

The federal government adopted these recommendations through a single law – the Canada Health Act (1984) – that replaced the Hospital Insurance and Diagnostic Services Act and the Medical Care Act. Under section 20 of the new law, the federal government was required to deduct (dollar-for-dollar) from a provincial government's share of the federal transfer the value of extra charges or user fees imposed by any physician or health facility in that province.

In addition to incorporating the four funding conditions – public administration, comprehensiveness, universality and portability – from its earlier laws, the federal government added a new funding condition – accessibility – that was intended to support the new penalty on extra charges and user fees. At the same time, however, the federal government made it clear that provinces which eliminated these fees within three years of the introduction of the legislation would have their deductions reimbursed at the end of that period. By 1988, user fees had been virtually eliminated for insured services under the Canada Health Act (Bégin 1988; Health Canada 2004).

While the five conditions of the Canada Health Act (enumerated in Table 2.2) started out as funding criteria, over time they have come to represent the principles and values that underpin Medicare policy for Canadians. After months of extensive national consultations in 2001 and 2002, the Commission on the

Table 2.2   Five funding conditions of the Canada Health Act (1984)

Condition	Each provincial health care insurance plan must:
Public administration Section 8	Be administered and operated on a non-profit basis by a public authority
Comprehensiveness Section 9	Cover all insured health services provided by hospitals, physicians or dentists (surgical-dental services which require a hospital setting) and, where the law of a province permits, similar or additional services rendered by other health care practitioners
Universality Section 10	Ensure entitlement to all insured health services on uniform terms and conditions
Portability Section 11	Not impose a minimum period of residence, or waiting period, in excess of three months for new residents; pay for insured health services for its own residents if temporarily visiting another province (or country in the case of non-elective services); and cover the waiting period for those residents moving to another province after which the new province of residence assumes responsibility for health care coverage
Accessibility Section 12	Not impede or preclude, either directly or indirectly, whether by charges made to insured persons or otherwise, reasonable access to insured health services

Sources: Canada Health Act 1984; Health Canada 2004.

Future of Health Care in Canada concluded that the five principles had "stood the test of time" and continued "to reflect the values of Canadians" (Canada 2002:60).

2.2   Organizational overview

Fig. 2.1 is a highly simplified organization chart illustrating the governance of public health care in Canada. Solid lines represent direct relationships of accountability, while dotted lines indicate more indirect or arm's-length relationships and influences.

Canada is a federal state with divided authorities and responsibilities determined by the constitution. With the exception of jurisdiction over hospitals and psychiatric institutions which the constitution assigns exclusively to the provinces, the authority over health or health care was never explicitly addressed in the original document that assigned powers to the central and provincial governments in the 1860s. As a consequence, authority can only be inferred from a number of other provisions in the constitution. Judicial interpretation of these provisions, as well as more general authorities on the constitution, support the view that the provinces have primary, but not exclusive jurisdiction over health care (Braën 2004; Leeson 2004).[6]

---

[6] Despite the fundamentally different constitutional status of the territories, they have been delegated "primary" responsibility for the health care of their residents by the federal government.

Fig. 2.1   Organizational overview

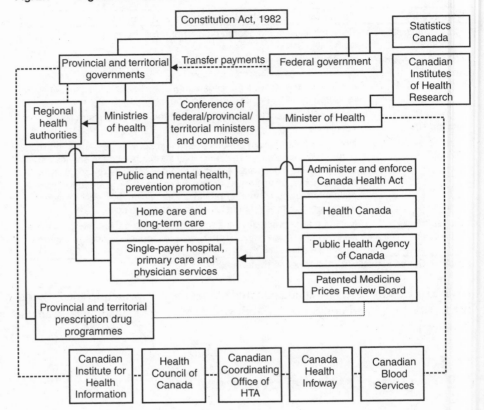

At the same time, the federal government, through its general powers, is responsible for protecting the health and security of Canadians. This, combined with the "spending power" (the ability of governments to spend in areas beyond their jurisdictional responsibilities), has permitted the federal government a role in setting the standards for the national Medicare system discussed above as well as to take up its responsibilities in public health, drug and food safety regulation and health research. The constitution also confers on the federal government the responsibility for health care for selected groups including First Nations people living on reserves and the Inuit, members of the armed forces, veterans, the Royal Canadian Mounted Police and inmates of federal penitentiaries.

2.2.1   The provincial and territorial level

Each province and territory has legislation governing the administration of a single-payer system for universal hospital and medical services. In addition to paying for hospitals, either directly or through global funding for regional health authorities, provinces also set rates of remuneration for physicians through fee schedules that are negotiated with provincial medical associations. Some specialized mental health and public health facilities and services are run directly by provincial departments of health.

By the late 1980s, a number of provinces were beginning to consider major reforms to the organization of their health delivery systems. Within a decade, most jurisdictions had established geographically based regional health authorities, a development reviewed in detail in section 7.

Provinces also provide, directly or indirectly, a variety of home care and long-term care subsidies and services. Finally, all provinces administer their own prescription drug plans providing varying degrees of coverage to residents.[7] These services have grown over time, and occupy a large part of provinces' resources. Fig. 2.2 illustrates the increase in the proportion of these non-Medicare public health services (including prescription drugs) compared to Medicare services from 1975 to 2004.

Figure 2.2   Relative share of provincial and territorial Medicare and non-Medicare public health care services, 1975 and 2004

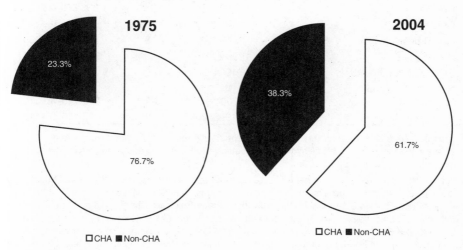

Source: CIHI 2004d.

Note: Figures for 2004 are forecasts. Since CIHI does not collect data using the Canada Health Act's (CHA) definition of medically necessary services, Medicare expenditures are estimated on the basis of hospital and physician expenditures, in effect a proxy for Medicare services made necessary by the current limitations in the data and its definitions.

---

[7] Prescription drugs provided in hospitals are treated as part of Medicare, whereas outpatient drug therapies are not, and as such are paid for out-of-pocket or through provincial prescription drug plans or private health insurance.

One of the objectives of regionalization was to improve continuity of care between the hospital and physician services with other, occasionally lower-cost and more appropriate, public health care services. Receiving global budgets from the province, regional health authorities (RHAs) are expected to allocate health resources in a manner that optimally serves the needs of their respective populations. They are also required to pay attention to the "upstream" health requirements of their populations with appropriate public health, illness prevention, health promotion programmes and activities. At the same time, no province has yet delegated RHAs the responsibility for the administration of prescription drug plans or physician remuneration (Lewis and Kouri 2004).

Table 2.3   Regionalization in provinces and territories, 1989–2005

Province or territory	Total population in thousands	Established/ changed (year)	Current number of RHAs	Population range of RHAs (2005)
British Columbia	4 196	1997/2001	5 (16)[a]	1 314 635–285 560
Alberta	3 202	1994/2003	9	1 042 855–66 005
Saskatchewan	995	1992/2001–2002	13	272 195–2 125
Manitoba	1 170	1997–1998/ 2002	11	622 015–955
Ontario	12 393	2005	14[b]	1 356 500–234 000
Quebec	7 543	1989–1992/ 2003	18	1 782 835–9 600
New Brunswick	751	1992/2002	8	179 840–29 325
Nova Scotia	937	1996/2001	9	398 038–33 165
Prince Edward Island	137	1993–1994/ 2005	0	–
Newfoundland and Labrador	517	1994/2003–2004	6/4/2[c]	295 145–40 516
Northwest Territories	43	1997–1998/ 2002	8	18 115–2 441

Sources: Lewis and Kouri (2004). Canadian Centre for Analysis of Regionalization and Health, updated provincial tables: http://www.regionalization.org/Regionalization/Reg_Prov_Overview_Table.html, accessed 3 July 2005.

Notes: [a] British Columbia's original 52 health authorities were made up of 11 regional health councils, 34 community health councils and 7 community health services societies. In 2002, this was restructured into 5 regional health authorities that administer a total of 16 health service delivery areas, as well as one provincial health authority responsible for province-wide services. [b] In 2005, the Government of Ontario established 14 local health integration networks. [c] In 1994, the Government of Newfoundland introduced a parallel structure for institutional and community care through 6 institutional health boards and 4 health and community services boards as well as 2 integrated boards. In 2002, the government announced its intention to create a modified structure that would further integrate institutional and community care services but it has not yet been implemented.

Provincial governments, directly as well as through RHAs and municipalities, provide an array of public health services. Many provinces have also initiated health information networks to improve the dissemination of clinical information on behalf of health providers and patients. Some provincial governments are also heavily involved in the assessment of health technologies as well as the funding of health research.

2.2.2   The federal level

While the provinces have the primary responsibility for the funding, administration and delivery of health care, the federal government plays a critical role in health research, data collection, public health and health protection. For constitutional reasons, it is directly responsible for the funding, administration and delivery of services to First Nations people and Inuit, war veterans, members of the Canadian armed forces and the Royal Canadian Mounted Police, and inmates of federal penitentiaries. It has also used its "spending power" through federal transfers to assist the provinces and territories in delivering public health care services in return for which provinces and territories agree to comply with a few basic conditions or principles that are contained in the federal law known as the Canada Health Act.

The federal department of health, Health Canada, is responsible for a number of activities including the (non-price) regulation and safety of therapeutic products (medical devices and drugs), as well as food and natural health products. In this regard, Health Canada approves drug products for sale in Canada based on the safety, quality and effectiveness of the products under the federal Food and Drugs Act. Health Canada is also a major funder of a number of arm's-length intergovernmental initiatives including the Health Council of Canada, Canada Health Infoway and the Canadian Patient Safety Institute.

Through its First Nations and Inuit Health Branch, Health Canada is responsible for community health programmes on First Nations reserves and in Inuit land claims areas, administering the non-insured health benefits (NIHB) programme for First Nations people and Inuit, and the funding and administration of public health and health promotion initiatives for First Nations people living on reserves, and Inuit throughout Canada. A sizeable proportion of funding and administration has been transferred to First Nations and Inuit groups through self-government agreements. The ministry is also responsible for various population health programmes including a major tobacco control initiative.

The federal Minister of Health is also responsible to Parliament for the Canadian Institutes of Health Research, the Patented Medicine Prices Review Board and the Public Health Agency of Canada as well as highly specialized agencies (not shown in Fig. 2.1) such as the Hazardous Materials Information Review Commission that deals with the use of potentially dangerous materials in industry as well as assisting in the protection of trade secrets in the chemical industry.

In 2000, the Canadian Institutes of Health Research (CIHR) supplanted the Medical Research Council as the country's national health research funding agency. The CIHR is made up of 13 "virtual" institutes with different focuses, as follows: Aboriginal peoples' health; ageing; cancer research; circulatory and respiratory health; gender and health; genetics; health services and policy research; human development, child and youth health; infection and immunity; musculoskeletal health and arthritis; neurosciences, mental health and addiction; nutrition, metabolism and diabetes; and population and public health. While the majority of CIHR-sponsored research is investigator-driven, approximately 30% of CIHR-funded research is based upon strategic objectives as defined by the governing council of CIHR. Overall, CIHR is part of the Government of Canada's stated objective of becoming one of the five leading health research nations in the world.

This research activity is supported by an extensive infrastructure for health data provided by Statistics Canada through the census as well as health surveys. Long known as one of the world's premier statistical agencies, Statistics Canada has been a pioneer in the gathering of health statistics as well as the development of indicators of health status, health resources (and their use) and the determinants of health. Data collection has been extended considerably through Statistics Canada's partnership with the Canadian Institute for Health Information (see section 2.2.3).

The federal government also provides the majority of funding for some major research initiatives that are conducted independently of the federal government such as Genome Canada and the Canadian Health Services Research Foundation (CHSRF). Genome Canada is the primary funding and information resource agency in the country. With its five genome centres spread out from British Columbia to Atlantic Canada, Genome Canada's objective is to make Canada a world leader in research that can identify a predisposition to disease as well as develop better diagnostic tools and prevention strategies. CHSRF focuses on research and dissemination in health services that is aimed at improving health organization, administration and delivery in the country as well as acting as a knowledge broker between the research community and health care managers, policy-makers and decision-makers.

In 1987, the Government of Canada first established the Patented Medicine Prices Review Board (PMPRB) to act as a watchdog on patented drug prices at the same time the patent protection for pharmaceuticals was enhanced. An independent, quasi-judicial body, the PMPRB regulates the "factory-gate" price, rather than retail price, of patented drugs – the price at which a drug manufacturer sells to hospitals, pharmacies and other wholesalers. Although the PMPRB has no mandate to regulate generic drug prices, it does report annually to Parliament on the price trends of all drugs.

Established as a departmental entity in 2004, the Public Health Agency of Canada performs a broad array of public health functions. These include surveillance, emergency preparedness, infectious disease control, national immunization and vaccines as well as national initiatives addressing injury prevention, chronic diseases and travel health. As part of its mandate, the Public Health Agency of Canada is responsible for the following regionally- distributed centres and laboratories:

- Centre for Healthy Human Development
- Centre of Chronic Disease Control and Prevention
- Centre for Infectious Disease Prevention and Control
- Centre for Emergency Preparedness and Response
- Centre for Surveillance Coordination
- Laboratory for Foodborne Zoonoses
- National Microbiology Laboratory

2.2.3   The intergovernmental level

As a decentralized state operating in an environment of increasing health policy interdependence, the provincial, territorial and federal governments rely heavily on both direct and arm's-length intergovernmental instruments to facilitate and coordinate policy and programme areas (O'Reilly 2001). The direct instruments are federal/provincial/territorial (F/P/T) advisory councils and committees that report to the Conference of F/P/T Deputy Ministers of Health which in turn report to the Conference of F/P/T Ministers of Health. The intergovernmental instruments, some of which have been established very recently, include intergovernmental not-for-profit corporations as well as some nongovernmental not-for-profit agencies funded by the sponsoring governments.

The Conference of F/P/T Ministers of Health is co-chaired by the federal Minister of Health and a provincial Minister of Health selected on a rotating basis. This committee is mirrored by the Conference of F/P/T Deputy Ministers of Health with an identical chair arrangement. In order to conduct their work in priority areas of concern, the ministers and deputy ministers of health have established, reorganized and disbanded various advisory committees over time. As of 2004, the following four advisory committees report to the Conference of F/P/T Deputy Ministers of Health:

- Advisory Committee on Health Delivery and Human Resources
- Advisory Committee on Population Health and Health Security
- Advisory Committee on Information and Emerging Technologies
- Advisory Committee on Governance and Accountability

In addition, the Conference of F/P/T Deputy Ministers of Health has authorized the creation of special task forces as well as working subcommittees and task groups under the advisory committees on issues of pressing concern to all jurisdictions. Finally, the Conference of F/P/T Deputy Ministers of Health appoints one of their members to act as liaison with the following intergovernmental agencies:

- Canada Health Infoway Inc.
- Canadian Coordinating Office for Health Technology Assessment
- Canadian Council for Donation and Transplantation
- Canadian Health Services Research Foundation
- Canadian Institute for Health Information
- Canadian Patient Safety Institute
- Health Council of Canada

Many of these intergovernmental agencies have been created recently. All are non-profit organizations with representatives from sponsoring governments sitting on their governing boards. In all cases, the federal government provides a significant share of the funding and in some cases almost all of the funding for their operations.

The Canadian Coordinating Office for Health Technology Assessment (CCOHTA) was first established in 1989. After a three-year trial period, CCOHTA was made a permanent, not-for-profit organization. Its mandate is to encourage the appropriate use of health technology by influencing decision-makers through the collection, analysis, creation and dissemination of analyses concerning the effectiveness and cost of technology and its impact on health (see *section 4.2.1*). Given the existence of provincial health technology assessment organizations, this also means that CCOHTA coordinates the dissemination of existing studies throughout the country as well as providing original health technology assessments in areas not covered by the provinces. CCOHTA is funded by Health Canada and, in proportion to population, by the provinces and territories (with the exception of Quebec which is not a member, in part because of its own considerable health technology infrastructure).

CCOHTA also examines both the clinical effectiveness and the cost-effectiveness of medical devices and drugs in an effort to extend and improve evidence-based decision-making, and is currently responsible for the Common Drug Review (CDR). The CDR is a single national alternative to separate provincial processes for reviewing new drugs. Since it began in 2003, all participating provinces and territories consider the CDR analyses in determining whether to include the pharmaceuticals reviewed in their respective formularies.

The Canadian Institute for Health Information (CIHI) was established in 1994 in response to the desire of the provinces, territories and central government for a nationally coordinated approach to gathering and analysing health information. Its core functions include: identifying national health indicators, coordinating the development and maintenance of national information standards, developing and managing health databases and registries, conducting research and analysis, and disseminating health information.

F/P/T ministries of health as well as individual health care institutions provide funding for CIHI. CIHI also has an ongoing working relationship with Statistics Canada, and many of its publications are co-sponsored by Statistics Canada. CIHI's 16-member board of directors has a strong advisory relationship with the Conference of F/P/T Deputy Ministers of Health. Although the Government of Quebec is not a formal member of CIHI, it does collaborate with and have observer status in the organization.

Canada Health Infoway is a product of the 2000 First Ministers' Accord on Health Care Renewal and the commitment of the F/P/T ministries of health to accelerate the development of electronic health information using compatible standards and communication technologies. In the 2003 First Ministers' Accord on Health Care Renewal, Infoway received further funding plus an expanded mandate to support telehealth development in Canada. Infoway acts as a national umbrella organization to facilitate the interoperability of existing F/P/T electronic health information initiatives as well as a catalyst for developing a pan-Canadian infostructure within an accelerated time frame. In 2003, Infoway released a common framework and standards blueprint for electronic health record development (Canada Health Infoway 2003). All F/P/T deputy ministers of health, including that of Quebec who joined in 2004, are members of Infoway.

The origins of the Health Council of Canada can be found in the final recommendations of the Romanow Commission and the Senate Committee, although the general idea of creating an intergovernmental body with some functional independence from the F/P/T ministers and deputy ministers of health has a longer history (Canada 2002; Senate 2002a; Adams 2001). After much intergovernmental discussion and disagreement, the Health Council was established without the participation of the provinces of Quebec and Alberta. The board of the Health Council is chaired by an individual nominated by consensus of the participating F/P/T ministers of health. The remaining 26 members of the board are based on the nominations of each jurisdiction, half of whom are direct representatives of F/P/T governments and the other half selected by F/P/T ministers of health as representatives of the general public as well as the expert community.

The Health Council of Canada's mandate is to monitor and report on the implementation of the 2003 first ministers' health agreement, particularly its accountability and transparency provisions (CICS 2003). This mandate was extended by the first ministers to include reporting on the progress of their 2004 *Ten-Year Plan to Strengthen Health Care* (CICS 2004). In its first report, the Health Council of Canada covered a broad set of issues including Aboriginal health, patient safety, primary care, home care, pharmaceutical management, waiting times, human resources, information technology and the development of comparable health indicators (Health Council of Canada 2005).

Canadian Blood Services (CBS) is a not-for-profit charitable organization that was created by the provinces and territories in the late 1990s in response to the tainted blood controversy and the exit of the Canadian Red Cross from the management of blood and blood services in Canada (Rock 2000). Although funded by the participating provinces and territories, Canadian Blood Services operates at arm's-length from all governments. While the agency's board members are nominated by provincial/territorial ministers of health, government representatives are not permitted on the board. Quebec has created its own blood and blood products management agency – Héma-Québec.

The Canadian Patient Safety Institute (CPSI), with its head office in Edmonton, Alberta, was established in December 2003. The creation of this institute was the key recommendation in a report by the nongovernmental National Steering Committee on Patient Safety (2002). The CPSI has stakeholder and government representatives on its board of directors. Its mandate is to disseminate models of best practice aimed at improving patient safety as well as to advise health system managers to initiate change that will support major patient safety improvements.

2.2.4   Nongovernmental national agencies and associations

Canadian health care programmes and policies are highly influenced by a number of nongovernmental agencies including health-service agencies and associations, charities, health professional associations and unions, health professional regulatory colleges, and private research institutes. Many are organized within individual provinces. A recent study found 244 such nongovernmental organizations operating in Ontario alone (Wiktorowicz et al. 2003). Some of these provincial organizations have national umbrella organizations that play an important role in facilitating and coordinating pan-Canadian initiatives. Some of the larger or more influential of these national organizations are described below.

The Canadian Council on Health Services Accreditation (CCHSA) is a voluntary, nongovernmental organization that accredits a number of hospitals and health facilities. Funded by the organizations it accredits, CCHSA also conducts reviews and assessments of health facilities or organizations with recommendations for improvement. CCHSA grew out of the Canadian Council on Hospital Accreditation, which was first established in 1958. Over time, CCHSA expanded its mandate beyond acute care hospitals to mental hospitals (1964), long-term institutions (1978), rehabilitation facilities (1985), community and comprehensive health services (1995), and home care services (1996).

Health provider organizations, particularly physician organizations, and in more recent decades, nurse organizations, have played a major role in shaping public health care policy in Canada. Other provider organizations including those representing dentists, optometrists, pharmacists, psychologists, radiologists, technologists and many others are now demanding a greater say in future public health care developments (Naylor 1986; Canada 2002; Romanow and Marchildon 2003).

The Canadian Medical Association (CMA) is the umbrella national organization for physicians, including specialists and general practitioners. In addition to lobbying for its members' interests, the CMA also conducts an active policy research agenda and publishes the biweekly *Canadian Medical Association Journal* as well as six more specialized medical journals. The 12 provincial and territorial medical associations (Nunavut is not represented) are self-governing divisions within the CMA. Except in Quebec where negotiations are carried out by two bodies representing specialists and general practitioners, these provincial and territorial bodies are responsible for negotiating physician remuneration and benefits with provincial governments. While the CMA is not involved directly in such bargaining, it does (when called upon) provide advice and expertise to the provincial associations on a host of topics ranging from remuneration to intergovernmental positioning.

The role of the CMA and, in particular, its provincial divisions, must be separated from the regulatory role of the provincial colleges of physicians and surgeons. The latter are responsible for the licensing of physicians, the development and enforcement of standards of practice and the investigation and discipline of physicians concerning standards of practice or for breaches of ethical and professional conduct. As is the case with most professions within Canada, physicians are responsible for their own regulation within the framework of provincial legislation. The Royal College of Physicians and Surgeons of Canada restricts its function to overseeing (and regulating) postgraduate medical education.

The Canadian Nurses Association (CNA) is a federation of 11 provincial and territorial registered nurses associations with approximately 120 000 members. Some of these provincial organizations such as the Registered Nurses Association of Ontario (RNAO) carry considerable political influence within their jurisdictions. The CNA and its provincial affiliates have played a major role in carving out a larger role for nurse practitioners in the health system (CNA 2003).

Unlike the CMA's provincial divisions, however, the provincial nurses associations are not involved in collective bargaining with the provinces. This is the function of the various provincial unions representing registered nurses (RNs), and licensed practical nurses (LPNs). The Canadian Federation of Nurses Unions is an umbrella organization for every provincially based nurses' union with the exception of Quebec.

Other citizen-based health care groups mobilize support and funding for their respective causes such as (but not limited to) the Canadian Healthcare Association (formerly the Canadian Hospital Association), the Canadian Health Coalition, the Canadian Association of Retired Persons (CARP), the Canadian Public Health Association, the Canadian Women's Health Network, the Canadian Home Care Association, the Canadian Hospice Palliative Care Association and the Canadian Naturopathic Association. Other voluntary organizations exist to address what their members perceive to be serious deficiencies in the current system in addressing mental health, cancer, multiple sclerosis and Alzheimer's disease, among many others.

Finally, there are lobby groups that represent private-for-profit interests in health care, including (but again not limited to) the Canadian Drug Manufacturers Association, Canada's Research-Based Pharmaceutical Companies, the Information Technology Association of Canada, the Canadian Life and Health Insurance Association and the Insurance Bureau of Canada.

2.3   Patient rights, empowerment and satisfaction

Beyond the entitlement of Canadians to public health insurance coverage as defined under the Canada Health Act, general patient rights are not defined under any federal law or charter (Shushelski 1999). The question has arisen, however, whether section 7 of the Charter of Rights and Freedoms – "right to life, liberty and security of the person" – encompasses a right of access to health care within a reasonable time (Jackman 2004; Greschner 2004). Recently, the Senate Committee reviewing the federal role in health care recommended in favour of health care guarantees in terms of minimum waiting times that should be promulgated and presumably enforced by the federal government (Senate 2002a).

However, it is unlikely that the federal government is ever going to legislate a set of health care guarantees on timeliness and quality. In addition to being difficult to monitor, such federal guarantees would probably intrude on the constitutional responsibility of the provinces to administer and deliver health care. More importantly, the recent Supreme Court of Canada decision in *Chaouilli* v. *Quebec (see section 8.2)* may push provinces and territories to do everything possible to limit their legal exposure including avoiding explicit patient charters or precise pronouncements on minimum waiting times for given procedures.

Outside special areas such as abortion and care of the elderly, there has been no general patient rights organization in Canada. Despite this, there is growing pressure on governments to ensure more patient-centred delivery, and a number of reform efforts are taking into consideration patient interests and expectations. This is partly due to the sensitivity of governments to growing patient dissatisfaction during the 1990s.

During and following the cuts to public health care budgets by both orders of governments, Canadians became increasingly anxious about the quality of the health care system as a whole. Table 2.4 illustrates this decline over the 1990s in response to the survey question: "Thinking broadly about Canada's health care system and the quality of medical services it provides, how would you describe it overall?" More recent survey evidence indicates that Canadians' concerns about the capacity of their public system's ability to deliver timely access to quality care peaked in the late 1990s and they continue to support publicly financed and administered systems even if they are divided on the issue of private-for-profit delivery within that system (Abelson et al. 2004).

Table 2.4   Canadians' perception of overall quality of the health care system, 1991–2000

	1991	1993	1995	1996	1998	1999	2000
Excellent/very good	61%	55%	41%	40%	30%	28%	29%
Good	25%	29%	30%	31%	38%	32%	34%
Fair/poor/very poor	12%	13%	15%	21%	32%	41%	34%

Source: Mendelsohn 2002.

Waiting times for surgery, diagnostic services and access to physicians have fuelled some of this dissatisfaction. While there is much debate concerning the nature and impact of waiting lists in Canada, it became one of the major themes in the First Ministers' Meeting on the Future of Health Care in September 2004 (CICS 2004). In addition, the Canadian Medical Association has encouraged provincial and territorial governments to move towards minimum treatment time protocols (CMA 2005), although they may be reluctant to move in this direction if they feel that this increases their exposure to litigation.

3. Financial resources

The principal source of health care finance is taxation by the provincial, territorial and federal governments. The remainder comes from individual patients in the form of out-of-pocket payments and private health insurance. This money is allocated to health organizations and providers primarily by governments for a host of health services and goods that are provided or subsidized by governments and, secondarily, by individual patients and consumers for a number of health goods and services that are in the private sector. Fig. 3.1 outlines the flow of resources in the Canadian health system.

3.1 Revenue collection

Approximately 70% of total health expenditure is financed from taxation by the provincial, territorial and federal governments. Private payment is split between out-of-pocket payments and private health insurance, with the former making up 15%, and the latter 12%, of total health expenditures. The remaining 3% of expenditure comes from a number of heterogeneous sources including social insurance funds, mainly for health benefits through workers' compensation, and charitable donations targeted to research, health facility construction and hospital equipment purchases (CIHI 2004d).

There have been some important shifts in revenue mobilization for health over time. Public sector revenue sources have declined relative to private sector revenue sources, with the most rapid increase in the ratio of private to public sector investment occurring during the first half of the 1990s – a direct result of provincial expenditure restraints. Table 3.1 shows the sources of health expenditure from 1975 to 2004.

In terms of the private sector, the changes have been more dramatic. Since 1988, the proportion of private health insurance relative to out-of-pocket expenditures has increased dramatically, from less than 30% to slightly more

Fig. 3.1   Financial flows

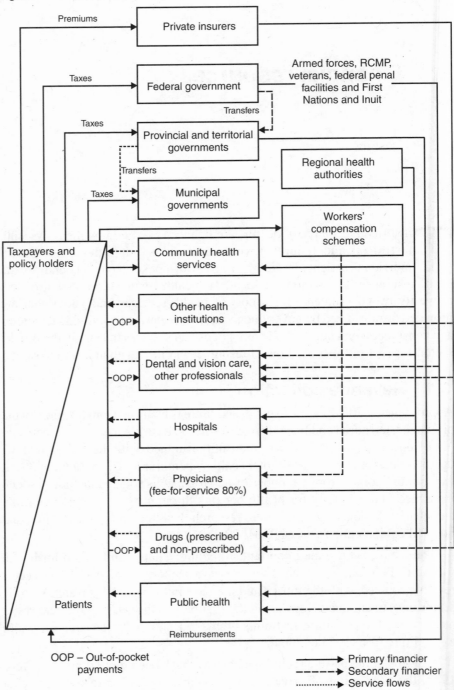

OOP – Out-of-pocket
payments

——————▶ Primary financier
–––––▶ Secondary financier
··············▶ Service flows

Fig. 3.2   **Percentage of total expenditure on health by source of revenue, 2002**

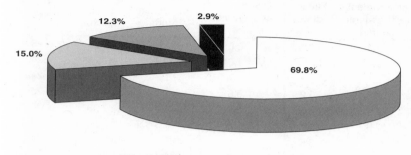

☐ Taxation ▨ Out-of-pocket ▨ Private insurance ■ Other

Source: CIHI 2004d.

Note: The "other" component of the private sector includes non-patient revenue to hospitals including ancillary operations, donations, investment income, etc.

than 40% of total private expenditure, whereas out-of-pocket revenues have dropped from 58% to slightly less than 50% of private finance (see Table 3.2). While the reason for this shift is probably to be found in escalating prescription drug costs and the corresponding growth in private health insurance, and the extent to which such costs are covered under private health insurance, this shift and its implications remain largely unexamined.

3.1.1   Compulsory sources of finance

The dominant sources of funding are the general revenue funds (GRF) of provincial and federal governments, the bulk of which come from individual income taxes, consumption taxes and corporate taxes. In addition, some provinces raise supplementary health revenues through notionally earmarked taxes known as premiums. In Alberta and British Columbia, these premiums are in reality poll taxes. The same "tax" is imposed on individuals and families irrespective of utilization or income, although provincial residents with incomes below specified levels or receiving social assistance are exempt from part or all of this payment. This premium revenue is collected outside the regular income tax system.

In Alberta, the annual premium currently amounts to C$528 for a single person and C$1056 for a family, while in British Columbia it is C$648 for a single person, C$1152 for a couple of two and C$1296 for a family of three

Table 3.1   Total health expenditure (%) by source of finance, 1975–2004

	Provincial government (with federal transfers)	Federal direct	Municipal government	Social insurance funds	Total public sector	Private sector
1975	71.4	3.3	0.6	1.0	76.2	23.8
1980	70.8	2.6	1.0	1.0	75.5	24.5
1985	70.8	2.9	0.7	1.2	75.5	24.5
1990	69.6	3.2	0.6	1.1	74.5	25.5
1995	66.1	3.6	0.5	1.1	71.3	28.7
1999	64.8	3.7	0.6	1.3	70.5	29.5
2000	64.8	3.6	0.6	1.4	70.4	29.6
2001	64.2	3.8	0.7	1.4	70.1	29.9
2002	64.0	3.8	0.7	1.4	69.9	30.1
2003	63.8	3.9	0.7	1.4	69.9	30.1
2004	64.0	3.6	0.8	1.4	69.9	30.1

Source: CIHI 2004d.

Notes: 2003 and 2004 are forecasts only. The provincial government column also includes territorial government. "Federal direct" refers to federal government spending through Health Canada and agencies such as the Patented Medicine Prices Review Board and the Public Health Agency of Canada as well as expenditures in relation to health care services for special groups such as First Nations people and Inuit, the Royal Canadian Mounted Police, the armed forces and veterans, as well as expenditures for health research, health promotion and health protection that occur outside Health Canada. Federal direct health expenditure does not include general health transfer funding to the provinces and territories, nor does it include transfers by the federal department of Indian and Northern Affairs to the territorial governments for the medical care and hospital insurance plans on behalf of First Nations peoples and Inuit. Municipal government expenditures include public health and capital construction and equipment expenditures by cities as well as dental services provided by municipalities in Nova Scotia, Manitoba and British Columbia. Designated funds transferred by provincial governments to municipalities for health purposes are not included. Social insurance funds are social insurance programmes that involve compulsory contributions by employees, employers, or both, with the government authority determining the terms on which benefits are paid to recipients. These include health care spending by provincial and territorial workers compensation boards and the drug insurance fund component of the Government of Quebec's prescription drug programme.

or more. These rates are substantially higher than in the recent past and may reflect a growing trend towards this form of taxation.

In 2004, the Government of Ontario introduced a new health premium that is in fact an additional income tax or surtax. The tax is proportional to incomes that fall within five stepped income bands. The surtax is 0 for individuals with a yearly taxable income of less than C$20 000, and then moves up in steps from C$300 for incomes of C$25 000–36 000) to C$900 for incomes of C$200 600 and greater (McDonnell and McDonnell 2005). The Ontario premium is collected as part of the income tax system unlike the health premiums collected in Alberta and British Columbia.

Table 3.2 **Distribution of private sector health expenditures by source of finance, 1988 and 2002**

Source of finance	1988		2002	
	(C$ 000 000)	(%)	(C$ 000 000)	(%)
Out-of-pocket	7 435.3	58.1	17 136.5	49.7
Private health insurance	3 734.2	29.2	12 730.9	40.6
Non-consumption	1 625.9	12.7	2 941.6	9.7
Total expense	12 795.4	100.0	32 809.0	100.0

Source: CIHI 2004d.

Note: Non-consumption expenditure includes a number of heterogeneous components, such as hospital non-patient revenue, capital expenditures for privately-owned facilities and privately funded health research.

The importance of the premium as a revenue source varies among the three provinces that collect it but it forms, even with recent increases, a relatively small proportion of the total revenues collected for health. The recent MLA Task Force on Health Care Funding and Revenue Generation in Alberta (2002) concluded that premiums amounted to less than 13% of provincial health revenue needs compared to provincial taxation (70%) and federal health transfers (17%).

While most of the revenue raised by the federal government for health expenditures is transferred to the provinces, some is spent directly by the federal government on items such as public health, pharmaceutical regulation, drug product safety, as well as First Nations and Inuit health care services. These direct expenditures by the federal government have been growing relative to provincial government expenditures (including federal transfers) since the mid-1970s (see Table 3.1). This is due largely to increases in Aboriginal health expenditures. Transfer payments under self-government arrangements for First Nations and Inuit health alone amounted to over $625 million in fiscal year 2001/02 (Canada 2002).

A very small amount of health funding is raised through municipal taxation, largely for public health expenditures by cities. Unfortunately, there is a dearth of scholarly analysis of municipal public health expenditures in Canada.

The provinces depend upon own-source revenues for the bulk of their health expenditures. These revenues are supplemented by federal health transfers; however, the exact percentage of the federal contribution, and the manner in which it is calculated, have been a subject of considerable debate. Indeed, differing perceptions concerning the appropriate level of federal transfer and the degree of conditionality that has traditionally accompanied such transfers, have caused much intergovernmental conflict in recent years (Lazar and St-Hilaire 2004; Marchildon 2004b).

This confusion stems from the conversion of the original federal-provincial cost-sharing arrangements supporting Medicare to an overall transfer called Established Program Financing (EPF) in 1977. At that time, the cost-sharing formulation was altered in three ways. The first was the conversion of roughly half of the original cash transfer into a permanent tax point transfer. The federal government annually counts the value of this tax point transfer, while the provinces count only cash transfers. The second was the mixing of health transfers with federal transfers to provinces for postsecondary education. This created a problem in terms of calculating the allocation between health and other transfers over time. Third, after the decoupling of the transfers from Medicare, the provinces could use federal transfers for any expenditures generally defined as health, raising the question of whether the federal contribution should be calculated as a percentage of insured services under the Canada Health Act or as a percentage of total provincial health expenditures.

Introduced in 1995, the Canada Health and Social Transfer (CHST) further complicated matters by adding social assistance and social services to the general block transfer of postsecondary education and health. At the same time, the cash portion of the transfer was reduced and the automatic escalator clause eliminated, thereby triggering considerable intergovernmental acrimony as well as concerns about the impact of the changes.

The Commission on the Future of Health Care in Canada (the Romanow Commission) outlined the difficulties involved in calculating the federal share and provided its own estimates using both provincial/territorial health expenditures and estimated Canada Health Act expenditures as a denominator. Fig. 3.3 and Fig. 3.4 are updated estimates of the federal transfer contribution to the provinces using the Romanow Commission's allocation of the block transfer among health, postsecondary education and social assistance until 2004 when the federal government created a new Canada Health Transfer with a higher allocation for health relative to the two other social policy envelopes. From its nadir in 1998 the federal contribution to provincial/territorial funds has tended to rise since that time, and sharply as a consequence of the first ministers' agreements of 2003 and 2004.

The cash portion of the CHT flows to the provinces and territories on a per capita basis. Although arguments have been made in favour of population needs-based funding, there are major intergovernmental obstacles – primarily the opposition of wealthier provinces – to any major overhaul of the current transfer formula.

Fig. 3.3   Federal government transfers as a share of provincial/territorial health expenditures, 1989/1990 to 2005/2006 (billions of C$)

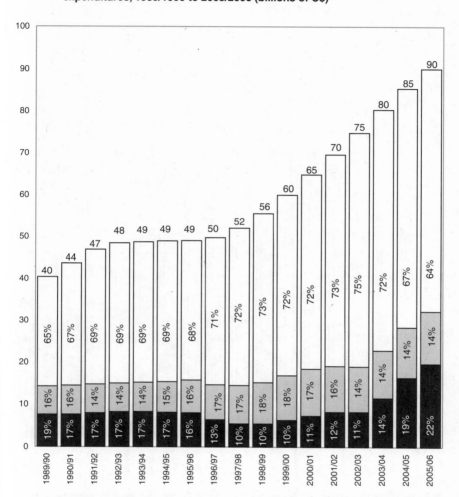

■ Federal cash transfers   ☐ Federal tax transfers   ☐ Provincial/territorial expenditures

Sources: Derived from: CIHI 2004d; Canada 2002; Finance Canada; Conference Board of Canada, 2004.

Notes: CIHI data are converted to "fiscal years" to allow for comparison with federal transfers for health. Estimates are applied to converted CIHI (2004e) data and Conference Board of Canada (2004) projections. The sudden jump in the percentage of the federal cash transfer in 2003/04 is a statistical result of assuming a 43% allocation in the block transfer before that date and the federal government's ultimate decision to allocate health 62% of the total block transfer when it created the Canada Health Transfer (CHT) in that year.

Fig. 3.4   Federal government transfers as a share of Canada Health Act services (billions of C$)

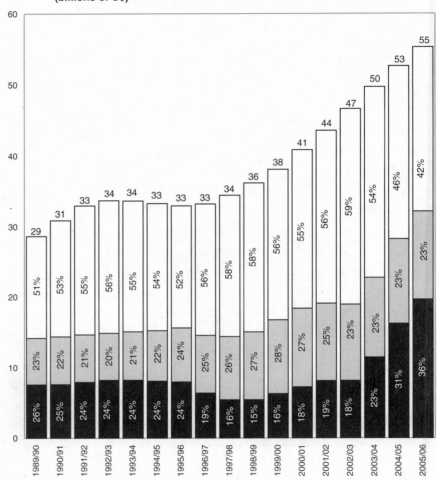

■ Federal cash transfers □ Federal tax transfers □ Provincial/territorial expenditures

Sources: CIHI 2004d; Canada 2002; Conference Board of Canada, 2004.

Notes: CIHI data are converted to "fiscal years" to allow for comparison with federal transfers for health. Estimates are applied to converted CIHI (2004e) data obtained and Conference Board of Canada (2004) projections. The 2003/04 increase in the federal cash transfer is exaggerated as a consequence of the 43% block funding allocation to health assumed before that date and the federal government's decision to allocate 62% of the original CHST block fund to health in that year with the creation of the CHT. Hospital and physician services have not grown at a rate comparable to other areas of provincial/territorial health expenditures (i.e. prescription drugs). As such, a 3-year average was used to derive the projected ratio of relative increase in total provincial/territorial expenditures to that of hospital and physician services.

3.1.2   Out-of-pocket payments

Constituting 15% of total health expenditure, out-of-pocket payments make
up the second most important source of funds for health care. Out-of-pocket
payments are the single most important source of finance for private health
goods and services. As shown in Table 3.2, however, this source of finance has
grown more slowly than private health insurance since the 1980s. Out-of-pocket
payments are the chief source of funding for vision care, over-the-counter
medication as well as complementary and alternative medicines and therapies
(Canadian Life and Health Insurance Association 2001).

3.1.3   Private health insurance

Private health insurance is the third most important source of funds for health
care in Canada constituting 12% of total health expenditure in 2002. In 2003,
53.6% of dental care, 33.8% of prescription drugs (worth C\$3.6 billion relative
to C\$5.5 billion for public insurance using 2001 data) and 21.7% of vision
care was funded through private health insurance. In contrast, Canadians hold
a limited amount of private health insurance for long-term care and home care
(Canadian Life and Health Insurance Association 2001; CIHI 2004d; Palmer
D'Angelo Consulting 2002).

Since the majority of private health insurance – particularly employment-
based insurance – is designed to provide coverage for health goods and services
not covered by Medicare, it can be classified as principally complementary in
nature (Mossialos and Dixon 2002). Private health insurance that attempts to
provide a private alternative, or faster access, to medically necessary hospital
and physician services is prohibited or discouraged by a complex array of
provincial laws and regulations. Six provinces – British Columbia, Alberta,
Manitoba, Ontario, Quebec and Prince Edward Island – prohibit the purchase of
private insurance for medically necessary services, although the prohibition in
Quebec has been called into question by the Supreme Court of Canada's ruling
in *Chaoulli* v. *Quebec* (see *section 8.2*). In the remaining four provinces, the
purchase of private insurance for such services is discouraged through various
means, such as preventing physicians who have opted out of the public plan from
charging more than the public fee schedule (Flood and Archibald 2001).

Most private health insurance comes in the form of group-based benefit plans
that are sponsored by employers, unions, professional organizations and similar
organizations (Canadian Life and Health Insurance Association 2001). Since this
type of insurance "comes with the job", it is not optional or "voluntary" health
insurance (VHI) as often described in many European countries (Mossialos and
Thompson 2004). Canadians receiving services through employment-based

private health insurance are exempt from taxation on these benefits except in Quebec where such benefits are now taxable under the provincial income tax regime. The federal Department of Finance estimated the value of non-taxation of business-paid health and dental benefits in Canada (minus Quebec) to be C$2.2 billion in 2004 (Finance Canada 2004).

3.1.4 Other sources of finance

Of the remaining heterogeneous sources of finance, the single most significant is social insurance funding from provincial workers' compensation schemes. Health benefits for work-related injuries under provincial workers' compensation plans pre-date the introduction of public health care with the first such scheme introduced by British Columbia in 1917. Administered by provincial workers' compensation boards (WCBs), these benefits are paid for by compulsory employer contributions that are set by provincial law (Association of Workers' Compensation Boards of Canada 2001). In 2003, WCB payments for health care services were estimated to be C$1.75 billion, which in turn constituted about 2% of public health care expenditures (CIHI 2004a). Much of this money is paid directly to provincial health authorities and individual health facilities for the provision of health services.

Health services provided through provincial and territorial WCBs are specifically excluded from the definition of insured health services under the Canada Health Act because they are funded under the authority of laws and administrative processes that pre-date provincial health insurance plans and federal health insurance legislation. As a consequence, WCB clients sometimes obtain – and are often perceived to be able to obtain – medically necessary services in advance of other Canadians, facilitated in part by WCB fees and payments to service providers that exceed Medicare rates. For this reason, the Romanow Commission suggested that this public form of queue jumping eventually be redressed through an intergovernmental reassessment of the health benefits portion of provincial WCB schemes (Canada 2002).

In 1997, the Government of Quebec established a social insurance drug plan funded through the compulsory payment of premiums by employers. The new law mandated that employers without a conforming drug benefit plan must introduce one, if they offered any form of private health insurance. At the same time, the provincial tax law was changed to make employee health benefits a taxable benefit thereby eliminating the tax expenditure subsidy for private coverage. At the same time, individuals without access to employment-based private health insurance (for example low-wage workers, retired persons and social assistance recipients) receive basic coverage from the provincial government (Palmer D'Angelo Consulting 2002). However, this basic coverage was also accompanied by new co-payments. In effect, these changes shifted costs from the provincial treasury to employers and employees as well as redistributing costs from taxpayers and patients.

Voluntary and charitable donations provide other sources of finance for health research as well as public health care. Numerous nongovernmental organizations – from hospital and disease-based foundations – regularly collect donations from the public. These funds are then used to purchase capital, equipment or research or to provide defined health services. Volunteers also donate their time and skills to various health service organizations. According to the Health Charities Council of Canada (2001), the voluntary sector raises and spends approximately C$300 million each year for health research.

3.2   Population coverage and basis for entitlement

Under the Canada Health Act (CHA), all residents of a province or territory are eligible to receive medically necessary services, without payment. This includes landed immigrants after an initial residency period (but not foreign visitors) as well as serving members of the Canadian military or Royal Canadian Mounted Police and inmates of federal penitentiaries. The last three groups are covered not by Medicare but by parallel federal public health insurance, although in practice provinces and territories simply charge the federal government for the provincial services used by members of these three groups. These medically necessary services, defined as "insured services" under the CHA, include virtually all hospital, physician (including some dental surgery) and diagnostic services (Health Canada 2004) as well as the primary care services offered under provincial Medicare plans.

Private insurance coverage for CHA-insured services is prohibited by provincial legislation in six provinces and discouraged through prohibitions of the subsidy of private practice by public plans in the other four provinces (see *section 3.1.3*). Contrary to popular belief, private provision of CHA-insured services is not illegal but providers are prohibited or discouraged from simultaneously operating in public and private domains (Flood and Archibald 2001). While private insurance for core CHA services is prohibited or discouraged by the provinces, they do permit a parallel public tier for health benefits, including some CHA services that are paid by provincial workers' compensation boards.

Although CHA-insured services are administered and provided by individual provinces and territories, their protection under federal legislation has, in the minds of many Canadians, elevated the status of insured services to entitlements or rights of Canadian citizenship. However, this sentiment has not been transformed into a substantial legal principle by the courts. Other health care services, including the many non-CHA services and subsidies provided by the provinces, are perceived more as benefits of residency rather than as rights or entitlements. First Nations people and Inuit are provided some additional benefits by the federal government, most notably non-insured health benefits (NIHBs) that go beyond what residents receive in most provincial and territorial public drug plans. These benefits include some extra prescription drug coverage as well as repayment for transportation costs incurred in seeking medical attention.

Since 53.6% of prescription drugs, 91.6% of vision care and 94.6% of dental care is funded privately, many Canadians use private health insurance (PHI) to cover part or all of the cost of these health goods and services. Currently, 33.8% of all prescription drugs, 21.7% of all vision care, and 53.6% of all dental care are funded through PHI (CIHI 2004d). Most of this insurance is employment-based and treated as part of compensation packages rather than privately purchased by individuals. At the same time, however, PHI is supported through substantial tax expenditure subsidies. Unfortunately, there has been little systematic study of the PHI sector in Canada.

3.3   Pooling agencies and mechanisms for allocating funds

Through the recent regionalization reforms in Canada (see *section 7*), the responsibility for the lion's share of financial resource allocation has shifted from health ministries to regional health authorities (RHAs) in most provinces and one territory. Each RHA is responsible for organizing a varying array of health and health care services and allocating a global budget for a designated population defined by a geographic area.

The funding method applied by individual provincial and territorial ministries of health varies across jurisdictions. Some provinces, particularly the western provinces, use a population-based funding method that attempts to evaluate the differing population health needs of each region, while others use more historically-based global budgets (McKillop, Pink and Johnson 2001; Hurley 2004).

RHAs are required to submit a budget to the appropriate provincial ministry of health. Most are required before the provincial or territorial budget is formulated and/or passed but in a minority of jurisdictions the RHA is required to submit a budget after general funding is announced by the province. Some provincial governments explicitly forbid RHAs from running deficits while others permit budget deficits under certain conditions (McKillop 2004). Yukon and Nunavut have not undergone regionalization, while Ontario is in the early phase of regionalization: in those jurisdictions, hospital and most other health facility funding is provided directly by the provincial government using various approaches (Senate 2002a).

3.4   Purchaser and purchaser–provider relations

The relationship between RHAs and the actual providers of health services combines relations based on hierarchical integration with relations based on contract. In this sense, RHAs act as both purchasers and providers. The majority of acute care facilities, including their salaried employees from nurses to technical support personnel, are managed directly by RHAs, although some RHAs do contract with some private providers for the provision of specialized ambulatory care services and a couple are considering similar arrangements for more comprehensive hospitals (CUPE 2004). As they are responsible for a defined population, RHAs are responsible for the "make or buy" decision.

Since all provincial governments continue to control physician budgets and manage prescription drug plans, the managerial scope of RHAs is constrained.[8] The vast majority of both specialists and general practitioners work under fee-for-service schedules and working arrangements that have been negotiated directly with the provincial ministry in a contractual relationship with RHAs and, as a consequence, specialists enjoy more autonomy relative to other health personnel within RHAs, while general practitioners operate largely outside the RHA system.

Nursing homes and other long-term care facilities are either run directly by RHAs or have a contractual relationship with RHAs. In reality, most RHAs have varying combinations of internally run facilities and independently run facilities with which they have an ongoing relationship. In the latter case, RHAs transfer an agreed-upon sum pursuant to a legal contract. A similar arrangement

---

[8] Dentists, chiropractors, optometrists and certain other health providers enjoy a degree of professional and organizational autonomy similar to physicians but, unlike physicians, largely operate outside the public health care system.

between an RHA and a contracted deliverer is also common in terms of certain home care, community care and palliative care services.

3.5   Payment mechanisms

There has been only limited study of payment mechanisms between provinces and RHAs, in part because of the very recent nature of regionalization reforms in Canada, including the more limited regionalization changes in Ontario (Hurley 2004). The major change initiated by these reforms is a shift from institution-specific funding (and to a much lesser extent, service-specific funding) to one based on comprehensive funding to organizations responsible for multiple health sectors with the freedom to allocate funds to each sector based upon the needs of a defined population (McKillop 2004). To answer the question of whether this has actually improved overall results in terms of efficiency, quality of care or population health requires further study. In addition, more research is required on the precise payment methods used by RHAs. In contrast to RHAs, health personnel remuneration – particularly physician fee-for-service – has been more extensively analysed.

3.5.1   Paying for hospital and clinical care

Most hospitals and clinics providing medically necessary services are allocated global budgets by regional health authorities.[9] Transfers to RHAs constitute the single largest item in provincial health budgets, and RHAs not only have the freedom to allocate their budget among various health organizations but also to determine the method of allocation and payment.

3.5.2   Paying health care personnel

Most health care personnel are paid salary to perform within hierarchically directed health organizations. Within this group, nurses – including registered nurses (RNs), licensed practical nurses (LPNs), psychiatric nurses and nurse practitioners – are the most numerous. Most general and specialist nurses are remunerated by way of salary based upon terms and conditions set by

---

[9] The health ministries in Yukon and Nunavut continue to fund hospitals directly through global budgets. Currently, the Ontario Ministry of Health and Long-Term Care provides global budgets to hospitals but the introduction of local health integration networks in 2005 may eventually shift the responsibility for budget allocation from the provincial government to these new regional authorities.

collective bargaining between the nurses' unions and province-wide employer organizations with the provincial government standing close behind. There is a growing use of temporary agencies for contracted nursing services for hospital and nursing home care, although this sector has not been examined systematically.

Nurse dissatisfaction with working conditions and stagnant remuneration during the provincial health reforms and budget cuts of the early to mid-1990s led to labour strife and rising absenteeism by the latter part of the 1990s. Since that time, nurse remuneration has improved as governments and health organizations have attempted to recruit nurses in a tight labour market (O'Brien-Pallas 2002; Zboril-Benson 2002; Canadian Nurses Advisory Committee 2002).

The majority of physicians continue to be remunerated on the basis of fee-for-service (FFS). There are some exceptions. Community clinic physicians, including physicians working within the Quebec community clinics (CLSCs) that were first created in the 1970s, are paid salary. More recently, some provinces have pursued alternative payment contracts with family/general practitioners, some of whom have accepted variations on a blended system of salary, capitation and FFS. For example, a remuneration model for family health networks has been developed in Ontario to provide incentives to promote preventive health care and chronic disease management (Ontario 2004). This model is based on: a capitated rate for all registered patients; FFS payments at a rate of 10% of the provincial schedule for most services; bonuses for targeted preventive care; payment for taking on new patients; continuing medical education allowances; some practice management fees; and some access to nurse practitioners remunerated by the government (Martin and Hogg 2004).

While many health policy analysts have been critical of the incentives created by FFS – including the incentive for overly rapid diagnosis and treatment – the system remains popular among many physicians and the organizations that represent them (Grignon et al. 2004). In the face of potential opposition as well as the international evidence indicating the negative incentives created by the alternatives, provincial governments have approached the reform of physician remuneration incrementally, and FFS payments continue to constitute approximately 83% of physician remuneration in Canada (CIHI 2004f). Table 3.3 provides the provincial division between FFS and alternative payment, although care must be taken as some provinces (for example, Manitoba) may classify physicians who receive part FFS and part alternative payment in the latter category only.

Alternative remuneration for physicians comes in many forms, only a few of which are, for example, connected to primary care reform. Based upon one provincial auditor-general's report, alternative payment seems to be concentrated

Table 3.3   Percent fee-for-service physician payment by province, 2002–2003

Province	Fee-for-service payment	Alternative payment
British Columbia	80.8%	19.3%
Alberta	91.4%	8.6%
Saskatchewan	86.6%	13.4%
Manitoba	64.1%	35.9%
Ontario	87.8%	12.2%
Quebec	77.4%	22.6%
New Brunswick	81.5%	18.5%
Nova Scotia	68.4%	31.6%
Prince Edward Island	78.5%	21.5%
Newfoundland and Labrador	63.3%	36.7%
Canada	**82.8%**	**17.2%**

Source: CIHI 2004f.

in specialties such as cancer care and psychiatry (British Columbia 2003). In other provinces, alternative payment contracts are provided to physicians for out-of-hours coverage of patients.

3.6   Health care expenditures

Of the estimated C$130 billion spent on health care in 2004, approximately 43% of total health expenditures were directed to hospital and physician services, the vast majority of which are considered medically necessary by the provinces and are therefore "insured services" under the terms of the Canada Health Act. A further 23% was spent on provincial programmes and subsidies for long-term care, home care, community care, public health and prescription drugs. An estimated 30% was spent on private health care services, a large portion of which was for dental and vision care services as well as prescription and over-the-counter drugs. Finally, roughly 4% was devoted to direct federal services including public health, the regulation of medicines, research and benefits for special groups including First Nations people living on reserves and Inuit (CIHI 2004d).

Like most OECD countries, Canada has experienced a growth in total health care expenditure (THE), measured as a percentage of GDP and as per capita increases in spending. Real annual growth in THE reached a peak in the late 1970s and the early 1980s, then declined precipitously in the early to mid-1990s only to rise again by 2000. In the early 1990s until 1997, real total health as well as real public health expenditure growth was substantially below real GDP growth reflecting severe public health expenditure cutbacks, producing a real (inflation-adjusted) decline in health spending. Throughout

Table 3.4   Trends in health expenditure, 5-year averages, 1976–2004

	1976–1980	1981–1985	1986–1990	1991–1995	1996–2000	2001–2004
Total health expenditure (THE) as % of GDP	7.0	8.0	8.5	9.6	9.0	9.9
Canada Health Act (CHA) services as % of THE	58.1	56.7	55.4	51.7	46.2	43.1
CHA services as % of GDP	4.1	4.5	4.7	5.0	4.2	4.3
Non-CHA services as % of THE	41.9	43.3	44.6	48.3	53.8	56.9
Non-CHA services as % of GDP	2.9	3.5	4.7	4.6	4.9	5.6
Mean annual growth rate in THE	12.8	12.4	8.9	4.0	5.8	7.4
Mean annual growth rate in CHA services	11.6	12.2	8.2	1.8	3.8	6.3
Mean annual growth rate in non-CHA services	14.6	12.7	9.8	6.3	7.5	8.2
Mean annual growth rate in GDP	12.6	9.1	7.0	3.6	5.8	4.7
Mean real annual growth rate in THE	3.3	4.2	4.0	1.6	4.0	5.0
Mean real annual growth rate in CHA services	2.2	4.0	3.3	-0.5	2.1	3.8
Mean real annual growth rate in non-CHA services	4.9	4.5	4.8	3.9	5.7	5.8
Mean real annual growth rate in GDP	3.6	3.1	2.3	2.0	4.3	2.2

Sources: CIHI 2004d; OECD 2004a; Statistics Canada 2004.

Notes: Hospital and physician expenditures are used as a crude proxy for Canada Health Act services since data are not collected on the basis of what provinces classify as Medicare services or publicly insure as medically necessary services. Real GDP figures are expenditure-based, seasonally adjusted, chained 1997 dollars. Real health expenditures are in constant 1997 dollars, calculated using the health component of the consumer price index (CPI). 2001–2004 is a four-year average.

this period, real growth in private health expenditures surpassed real growth in public health expenditures. By 1997, governments were beginning to reinvest in public health care, a trend that has continued to the present (CIHI 2004d). By 2003, the real growth in public health expenditures exceeded, by a small margin, the real growth in private health expenditures (Table 3.4).

During the 1970s and 1990s, the real growth in health expenditures was less than the rate of growth in the economy as a whole as measured by real GDP. The opposite was true during the 1980s and the first 4 years of the twenty-first century. Hospital and physician services, the proxy used for "insured services" under the Canada Health Act, have grown more slowly than other health services in the past three decades.

Fig. 3.5 **Health care expenditures as a share of GDP in Canada and selected countries, 1960 to 2002**

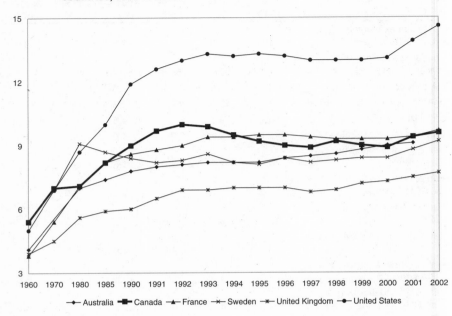

Source: OECD 2004.

The faster rate of growth of private health expenditures, and mixed public–private health expenditures, particularly for prescription drugs, has meant that total health expenditures have been growing as a percentage of GDP, eventually reaching 10% (CIHI 2004d). As illustrated in Fig. 3.5, this growth puts Canada in a very similar position to Australia, France and Sweden, with the United Kingdom devoting slightly less of its GDP to health care and the United States substantially more.

When examining public health care expenditures alone as a share of GDP (Fig. 3.6), a slightly different picture emerges. Here, Canada along with Australia, the United Kingdom and the United States is placed at the lower end, while France and Sweden both devote a substantially higher share of their respective GDPs to public sector health care expenditures. Both Canada and Sweden did experience a decline in public health expenditures in the early 1990s (Tuohy 2002; Hjortsberg and Ghatnekar 2001). In the case of Canada, public expenditure constraints were linked to the recession of the very early 1990s, the negative impact on government deficits and the decision by provincial governments, in particular, to address rising public debt through budget cuts.

Fig. 3.6   Public health care expenditures as a share of GDP in Canada and selected countries, 1960–2002

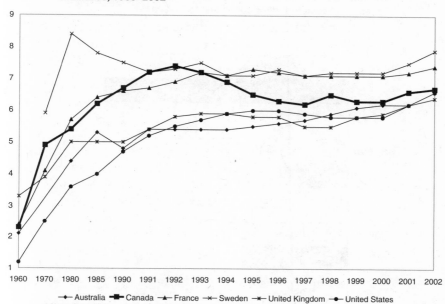

Source: OECD 2004.

Notes: Comparable OECD data are provided on a consistent annual basis by the 1990s. In some cases (United States and Australia) OECD data for earlier years are not available.

Examining health care expenditures as a share of GDP has serious limitations, the most important of which is the impact of recessionary periods in exaggerating the growth in health expenditures.

To avoid a measure that exaggerates the growth of health expenditures during a recession, health care expenditures can be calculated in terms of real per capita expenditures (Fig. 3.7). In addition, by separating public and private health expenditures, certain trends can be made clearer. Among the comparator countries, Canada and Sweden experienced the lowest rate of growth in public health expenditures from 1990 to 2001. It is also clear that the high growth rate in Canadian health expenditures was led by the private sector (in turn led by rising prescription drug costs), with Canada, next to Sweden, having the highest private health expenditure growth rate during the 1990s (Evans 2003).

As shown in Table 3.5, 30% of health expenditures are allocated to hospitals. Hospitals are defined as institutions licensed or approved as hospitals by provincial and territorial governments or operated directly by the federal government. Although hospitals mainly provide acute care, some comprehensive

**Fig. 3.7   Growth trends in real per capita health care expenditure, cumulative
percentage change in national currency units at 1995 GDP price level, in
Canada and selected other countries, 1990–2001**

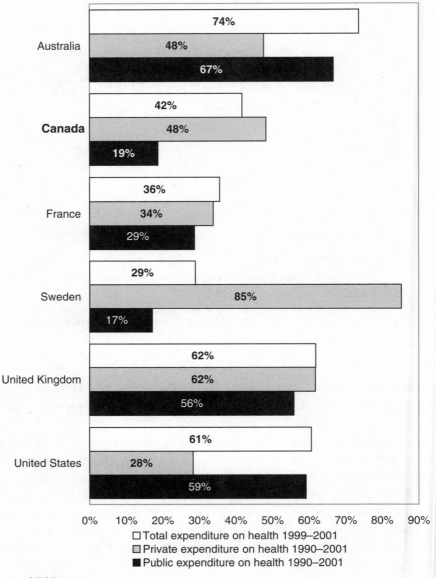

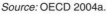 *Source:* OECD 2004a.

hospitals also provide some extended or chronic care, rehabilitation and convalescent care, and psychiatric care services. Hospitals also include nursing stations and outpost hospitals in remote areas.

Other institutions, defined as long-term care facilities for the chronically ill or disabled as well as residential facilities for persons with physical or psychiatric disabilities, emotional disturbances or alcohol and drug problems, now absorb 9.5% of total expenditures.

Table 3.5   Health expenditure by service category (% total health expenditures), selected years, 1975–2004

Year	Hospitals	Other institutions	Physicians	Other professionals	Drugs	Capital	Public health and admin.	Other health spending
1975	44.7	9.2	15.1	9.0	8.8	4.4	4.5	4.3
1980	41.9	11.4	14.7	10.1	8.5	4.4	4.3	4.6
1985	40.8	10.3	15.2	10.4	9.5	4.1	4.5	5.2
1990	39.1	9.4	15.2	10.6	11.4	3.5	4.2	6.7
1995	34.4	9.6	14.4	11.6	13.6	3.1	5.2	8.1
2000	31.2	9.5	13.3	11.8	15.4	4.0	6.4	8.4
2004[a]	29.9	9.6	12.9	11.2	16.7	4.5	6.7	8.6

Source: CIHI 2004d.

Note: [a] 2004 is a forecast.

Physicians are not included in hospital or other institutional expenditures. They constitute almost 13% of total health expenditures. This sector has been a relatively slow-growing segment of health care in Canada. Other professionals include dentists, optometrists, psychologists, chiropractors, massage therapists, denturists, orthoptists, osteopaths, physiotherapists, podiatrists, private duty nurses and naturopaths. The total share of this other professional segment is 11.9% of total health expenditures, of which roughly 60% is expended on dental services (CIHI 2004a).

Even larger than physician expenditures are drug expenditures – including both prescription drugs and over-the-counter drugs. Together, they constitute nearly 17% of total health expenditures. This is now the second largest category of health expenditures and the most rapidly growing segment of health care (both public and private) since 1975. This growth is largely due to the introduction of new prescription drugs since that time (CIHI 2004d; Evans 2003).

4.   Regulation and planning

4.1   Regulation

Canada has a highly decentralized health system with a mixed model of public and private health delivery. The provinces have primary jurisdiction over the administration and delivery of public health care services but "delegate" actual delivery to health organizations, as well as physicians working on fee-for-service schedules or mixed remuneration arrangements the terms of which are negotiated with the provincial governments. Health facilities and organizations, from the hospital to the regional health authority, are accredited on a voluntary basis through a nongovernmental organization. Most health care providers, including physicians, nurses, dentists, optometrists, chiropractors and psychologists, are organized as self-governing professions under provincial framework legislation.

4.1.1   Regulation and governance of third-party payers

In terms of public health care in Canada, the provinces are the principal third party payers. All provinces manage single-payer systems for the delivery of hospital, physician and diagnostic services. They also provide services and subsidies for prescription drugs, long-term care, home care, as well as public health, health promotion and illness prevention programming. As the principal payers, provinces work through, or contract with, a range of health care organizations and providers, from regional health authorities to individual hospitals and physicians.

In the provinces that are currently regionalized, a statutory relationship exists between provincial governments and regional health authorities in which the division of responsibility and accountability between the two is described in very general terms. In addition, some health authorities, such as the local health integration networks in Ontario, are subject to explicit performance agreements. However, the provincial Minister of Health and the provincial cabinet are ultimately accountable to all provincial residents for administering and delivering public health care and thus for the performance of regional health authorities.

In contrast to the provinces, the three territories are constitutionally and fiscally dependent on the federal government for the administration and funding of health care. In terms of health governance and administration, the federal government has, over time, delegated powers and responsibilities that are similar to those that the provinces hold. However, as a consequence of their inadequate tax base and the high cost of delivering services in the sparsely populated north, the territories are heavily reliant on federal fiscal transfers well beyond their per capita allocation under the Canada Health Transfer.

Under the constitution, the federal government is responsible for First Nations people living on reserves and Inuit. In recent decades, this responsibility has been gradually turned over to some First Nations and Inuit communities through a series of self-governing agreements covering community-based health care services, health promotion and illness prevention initiatives, and the administration of the Non-Insured Health Benefits (NIHB) Program (Health Canada 2003b).

For other Canadians, most dental, vision, chiropractic, psychological and naturopathic health care, as well as approximately one half of prescription drugs and virtually all complementary and alternative medicines, are funded and delivered privately. The main sources of funding for these services are user fees and private health insurance. Most private health insurance comes in the form of group insurance plans sponsored by employers, although some private health insurance is also sponsored by trade unions and professional associations. Unlike voluntary health insurance (VHI) in many European countries, private health insurance (PHI) in Canada is a compulsory portion of the benefits package for many employees.

The types of policies vary considerably in terms of benefits, but prescription drug benefits and dental care benefits constitute almost 80% of total private health insurance benefits payments in Canada (Canadian Life and Health Insurance Association 2001). Private health insurance also plays an important role in covering non-physician health providers such as psychologists, chiropractors, physiotherapists, podiatrists, osteopaths and optometrists. Both public health coverage and private health insurance exclude most types of complementary and alternative medicine (CAM), although some CAM provider services are covered under a minority of PHI policies.

All federally incorporated private health insurance companies are required to provide an annual financial statement to a federal regulator to ensure financial soundness. The provinces are responsible for regulating provincially incorporated health insurance companies and for regulating the conduct of all insurance agents as well as contractual matters related to consumer service.

4.1.2   Regulation and governance of providers

Providers fall into two groups: on the one hand, health institutions such as hospitals, nursing homes, health clinics and regional health authorities; and health professionals who are generally organized in self-governing professional bodies, on the other.

As discussed in section 2, historically the vast majority of hospitals were private, mainly not-for-profit institutions that operated at arm's-length from provincial governments, although some government regulation and supervision had long been accepted in return for subsidies and grants. With the introduction of hospitalization, however, the relationship between hospitals and governments became much closer, with hospitals almost entirely reliant on public funding through global budgets, and governments ultimately accountable for this use of public funds. With regionalization, hospitals have been drawn into an even closer relationship with provincial governments with many no longer governed by an individual board of directors.[10]

Despite the major shift towards a regionalized system of administration and delivery in most provinces, health facility accreditation through the Canadian Council on Health Services Accreditation remains voluntary and nongovernmental in nature. Health institutions and their providers, in particular physicians, are liable to patients for negligence. Lawsuits for medical malpractice and similar negligence based on tort law are pursued privately through the courts.

Damage awards and therefore malpractice insurance costs are not nearly as high in Canada as in the United States for a number of reasons. These include the more restricted practice of contingency billing by lawyers, damages that are awarded by judges rather than juries, and the policy of physician associations to fight rather than settle "nuisance" claims. Nevertheless, it is generally recognized that the incentives created by the private tort system can potentially impede health care reform as well as constrain government efforts to reduce health expenditures (Caulfield 2004; Mohr 2000).

---

[10] Quebec and Ontario are the important exceptions to this general trend. Some hospital boards also continue to operate in Manitoba.

There has been no major empirical study of medical malpractice in Canada since the Pritchard report commissioned by federal, provincial and territorial deputy ministers in the late 1980s (Pritchard 1990). Despite the serious problems associated with the private tort system, the Pritchard report none the less rejected the policy alternative of provincial governments moving to a no-fault compensation system, and medical malpractice through the private tort system remains the norm in all provinces and territories.

In the main, professional standards and codes of conduct are set through the relevant profession's regulatory body and the provincial laws that give the profession the right to self-regulate subject to certain terms and conditions. At the same time, these professional standards respond to the standards that are established judicially through medical malpractice litigation. Today, there are approximately 35 health professions that are self-regulated in this manner (CIHI 2001).

There are three different approaches to provider regulation in Canada. The first is "exclusive scope of practice", also known as licensure, where members of a profession are granted the exclusive right to provide a particular service to the public. The second is "right to title", also known as certification or registration, where members of a profession and non-members provide services to the public, but only members may use a protected title or describe themselves as being registered. The third is the "controlled acts system", in which a specific task or activity is regulated rather than the profession itself.

While the specific regulatory approach for provider groups can vary considerably from province to province, there is remarkable consistency in approach among certain professionals such as physicians and dentists. Moreover, there has been considerable intergovernmental work to address the issue of portability of qualifications among provinces (Casey 1999, CIHI 2001). Finally, some provinces have experimented with a single overall law that provides a common regulatory framework for all the health professions. In Ontario, for example, the Regulated Health Professions Act (1993) applies to the 23 health professions and the 21 colleges that regulate them. The common objectives of the law include: protecting the public from harm; promoting high quality care; making regulated health professions accountable to the public; giving provincial residents access to the health care professions of their choice; achieving equality by making all regulated health professions adhere to the same principles; and treating providers (and their patients/clients) equitably (Ontario 1999).

It is important not to confuse the function of professional self-regulation with the other roles performed by professional bodies. These may include a general advocacy role for the profession as well as the protective and advancement functions associated with collective bargaining concerning fee schedules, salaries and working conditions. In the case of physicians, the national and provincial medical associations are responsible for the latter functions and are separate from the national and provincial colleges that are responsible for regulating the profession. In the case of nurses, the national and provincial nursing associations are responsible for raising the professional profile, as well as improving nurse education and training, while nurses' unions are responsible for collective bargaining. In principle, these functions can, and should, be separated. In practice, however, they have occasionally been confused.

4.1.3   Regulation and governance of the purchasing process

Health providers offering public health care services can be employed directly by health institutions (whether an RHA or an individual health facility) or, like physicians, work under a fee schedule or general set of objectives, the terms and conditions of which are negotiated by the physicians' representative and the provincial government. Providers who are employees, such as nurses, work within hierarchical organizations, delivering services according to a pattern and pace established by the organization over time. Their performance is supervised by managers, some of whom are providers with management responsibilities. In contrast, fee-for-service physicians exercise more discretion in judgement and decision-making in the discharge of their professional responsibility than salaried – or even contracted – professionals.

Historically, Canada has depended heavily on internationally educated medical graduates. In the 1970s, roughly 30% of doctors practising in Canada were trained outside the country. While this number had declined to 22.5% by 2003, some low-population density jurisdictions with many rural and remote communities such as Saskatchewan (52.5%) and Newfoundland and Labrador (40.3%) continue to have an extremely high percentage of foreign medical graduates (CIHI 2004e).

Physicians trained abroad face a national examination set by the Medical Council of Canada as well as varying provincial licensing requirements before they can practise in Canada. At the same time, some provinces have introduced options for fast-track licensure of international medical graduates to alleviate shortages in particular areas (CIHI 2001).

In contrast to more mainstream health professionals, complementary and alternative medicine providers work in a less regulated environment. While a few are self-regulating through the conventional regulatory model, most are not, despite their considerable efforts to achieve provincial recognition with the "right to title" or "exclusive scope of practice". For example, while massage therapy is practised throughout Canada, it is only formally regulated in British Columbia and Ontario. Chinese medicine practitioners remain unregulated in most of Canada but are regulated in British Columbia (under the mandate of the College of Acupuncturists), the province where these services are most popular.

Beginning in 2004, the Natural Health Products Directorate of Health Canada has been regulating traditional herbal products, vitamins and mineral supplement and homeopathic preparations. These regulations include the initial approval of such CAM products as well as issues of labelling.

4.1.4   Purchase, regulation and governance of prescription drugs

Most prescription drugs are purchased by patients at the recommendation of family physicians. For the majority of these patients, the costs of prescription drugs are covered or subsidized by private health insurance or provincial/ territorial drug plans. Inpatient drug therapy is the exception. Since prescription drugs provided in hospitals are considered part of Medicare coverage, hospitals and regional health authorities do purchase in bulk but the amount purchased in this way is minor compared to prescription drugs purchased directly by outpatients. Based upon CIHI data for 2002, almost C$1.4 billion was expended on inpatient drugs. This was in addition to the C$6.4 billion spent by the provinces and territories on prescription drugs, almost all of which was through provincial drug plans (CIHI 2005).

Both orders of government are responsible for different aspects of the regulation and governance of prescription drug therapies. Through the Therapeutic Products Directorate (TPD) of Health Canada, the federal government determines the initial approval and labelling of all prescription drugs. However, since the provincial governments subsidize the purchase of prescription drugs, they deploy a number of cost containment strategies that include restrictive provincial formularies and reference pricing based on the lowest-cost (patented or generic) alternative. These provincial policies, particularly those that control choice of brand, along with provincial differences in consumption behaviours, are largely responsible for the variations in provincial drug spending (Morgan 2004).

Beyond this form of health and safety regulation, Health Canada also prohibits direct-to-consumer advertising of drug products and places some limits on the marketing of prescription drugs to physicians, although a large section of the Canadian public is nevertheless influenced by prescription drug advertising through cable and satellite television networks that originate in the United States (Mintzes et al. 2002).

The constitution confers exclusive jurisdiction over the patenting of new inventions, including new prescription drugs, to the federal government. The Patent Office is part of the Canadian Intellectual Property Office, a special operating agency associated with the federal department of Industry Canada.

In the late 1980s and early 1990s, the federal government changed its pharmaceutical policy direction by increasing patent protection to the OECD norm of 20 years and by abolishing compulsory licensing in a bid to increase the level of investment, research and development in Canada by the international pharmaceutical industry (Anis 2000). At this time, it created an arm's-length quasi-judicial federal body, the Patented Medicine Prices Review Board, to regulate the prices of patented drugs. On the other hand, due in part to its questionable constitutional authority, the federal government does not regulate generic drug prices (Menon 2001; Critchley 2002).

4.2   Planning and health information management

As a consequence of the constitution and the decentralized nature of health administration and delivery in Canada, there is no single national agency responsible for system-wide national planning. Instead, national initiatives are often the product of a series of intergovernmental committees and agencies that do a limited amount of planning on a sector-by-sector basis. The forum that is ultimately responsible for many of these planning initiatives is the Conference of F/P/T Ministers of Health and the Conference of F/P/T Deputy Ministers of Health.

In addition to the advisory committees and working groups established under this conference structure, arm's-length intergovernmental agencies have been established for planning, again on a sectoral basis. The most notable initiatives of this type include health technology assessment through the Canadian Coordinating Office for Health Technology Assessment (CCOHTA), health information and systems management through the Canadian Institute for Health Information (CIHI) and Canada Health Infoway, and comparable performance indicators through the Federal/Provincial/Territorial Advisory Committee on Governance and Accountability that reports to the Conference of F/P/T Deputy Ministers of Health.

Most system-wide planning is actually done within the ministries of health at the provincial level. Each provincial ministry has a policy and planning branch that provides regular advice on planning. Health evidence, information and systems management form an increasingly important part of the planning process with major initiatives and experimentation in a number of provinces. Some provinces have established health research agencies or health quality councils with a mandate to help the provinces improve health system outcomes. Using a different approach, Ontario established the Institute for Clinical and Evaluative Sciences (ICES) in order to influence physician practice and clinical decision-making.

To support system-wide planning, many provincial governments have also established health information technology infrastructures with plans to create personal electronic health records for all provincial residents. To varying degrees, this provincial planning is reinforced by the Advisory Committee on Information and Emerging Technologies, an intergovernmental committee that reports to the Conference of F/P/T Deputy Ministers of Health.

Perhaps the single most important initiative in system-wide planning has been the creation of regional health authorities (RHAs) by provinces. Operating at an intermediate level between health ministries and individual providers, RHAs have a planning mandate to improve the coordination and continuity of care among a host of health care organizations and providers within a geographic area (Denis 2004). While general framework planning is conducted at the provincial level, detailed planning and coordination, including health information systems, are actually done at the RHA level. RHAs set their priorities through annual budgets (occasionally supplemented by multi-year plans) that are submitted to provincial governments. Some budget submissions are required before the provincial budget is finalized while others are submitted only after funding is announced in the provincial budget, with each approach having a different consequence in terms of the planning process (McKillop 2004).

4.2.1   Health technology assessment

Objective and reliable health technology assessment (HTA) is essential to effective planning as well as evidence-based decision-making by health managers and providers. Since most technological progress is incremental, new advances tend to build directly on existing ideas, products and techniques. At the same time, however, there will be some unexpected leaps in health care technology that will have important implications in terms of both clinical effectiveness and cost of treatment. A recent example of the latter involves genetic testing and gene patenting (Giacomini, Miller and Browman 2003; Ontario 2002). HTA must deal with both types of technological change (Morgan and Hurley 2004).

According to one European observer, HTA organizations in Canada are now among the best-established in the world (McDaid 2003: 205). These agencies operate at both the provincial and intergovernmental levels. The first fully-fledged HTA agency, the Agence d'Évaluation des Technologies et des Modes d'Intervention en Santé (AETMIS) was established in Quebec in 1988. This was followed by provincial HTA agencies in British Columbia (since scrapped), Alberta, and Ontario. In the latter case, the Ontario Health Technology Advisory Committee provides the Ontario Ministry of Health and Long-Term Care and provincial health care providers with advice regarding the uptake, diffusion and distribution of new health technologies and the abandonment of obsolete health technologies. While there are no specific HTA organizations in other provinces, the more broadly based research agencies in Saskatchewan, Manitoba and Newfoundland and Labrador do conduct a limited amount of HTA research, while the Therapeutics Initiative in British Columbia assesses prescription drugs in that province (Roehrig and Kargus 2003).

These efforts are coordinated, at least to a limited degree, by the Canadian Coordinating Office for Health Technology Assessment or CCOHTA. First established by the federal, provincial and territorial ministers of health in 1990, CCOHTA's objective was to provide evidence-based information on existing and emerging health technologies, defined as medical procedures, devices, systems or drugs used in the maintenance, treatment and promotion of health. CCOHTA has since set up a Canadian Emerging Technologies Assessment Program (CETAP) and a Common Drug Review (CDR).

First established in 2002, the CDR provides a single process for reviewing new pharmaceuticals and providing recommendations concerning formularies to all provinces and territories with the exception of Quebec. The CDR process has three stages. In the first stage, CCOHTA makes a systematic review of the available clinical evidence as well as the pharmacoeconomic data. In the second stage, the Canadian Expert Drug Advisory Committee (CEDAC) under CCOHTA makes a formulary listing recommendation. In the third and final stage, provincial and territorial health ministries make their own formulary and benefit coverage decisions based in part on the CEDAC recommendation but also on the basis of the decisions of their own drug formulary committees. Provincial decisions will also be influenced by the presence or absence of a significant pharmaceutical industry presence. In Canada, most of the pharmaceutical industry is concentrated in Quebec and Ontario.

4.2.2   Health information

As befits its federal character, Canada has a number of information systems in place for the collection, reporting and analysis of health data. At the provincial level, governments have been collecting detailed administrative data since the introduction of hospitalization and Medicare. At the federal level, Statistics Canada has been collecting health information through both the national census and periodic health surveys. Statistics Canada is governed by a legislative framework – the Statistics Act – that makes the provision of census data compulsory. At the intergovernmental level, the CIHI coordinates the collection and dissemination of health information and develops and maintains national information standards.

Privacy has emerged as a major issue in health data collection and dissemination during the past decade. The collection and use of personal health information – including dissemination and retention – are inherently privacy-intrusive activities in which judgements are constantly being made as to whether the public good of obtaining, analysing and using this information outweighs the potential intrusion on an individual's privacy.

Jurisdiction over health information is shared among federal, provincial and territorial government creating a patchwork of health information and privacy laws in the country. These laws address three issues – privacy, confidentiality, and security – sometimes in the same legislation, at other times in separate laws within the same jurisdiction.

At the federal level, four major laws govern privacy. The Personal Information Protection and Electronic Documents Act (known by the acronym PIPEDA) applies to personal health information that is collected, used, or disclosed in the course of commercial activities that cross provincial and territorial borders. The Privacy Act requires informed consent before information is collected or used. Within a strict legislative framework protecting personal confidentiality, the Statistics Act permits Statistics Canada to collect information through a census every five years as well as periodic surveys. At the same time, the Access to Information Act requires that public information held by governments or government agencies be made publicly available unless it is specifically exempted.

At the provincial level, most jurisdictions have legislation in place to protect privacy, and some have legislation that protects health information in particular. This latter development is, in part, a response to the public backlash that provincial governments experienced in their initial efforts to establish electronic health information networks. While privacy concerns about health records pre-dated such efforts, the potential use of electronic health records has highlighted these concerns.

4.2.3   Research and development

Effective health systems research is essential to health planning. This type of research occurs at the provincial and federal levels of government. At the federal level, one of the Canadian Institutes of Health Research (CIHR) – the Institute of Health Services and Policy Research – is devoted to funding research into health systems policy and planning. First established in 1997, the Canadian Health Services Research Foundation (CHSRF) is an arm's-length national research organization whose central mandate is to improve the use of health services research by health system managers. A number of provincial funding organizations have also been established to encourage similar research to improve both health planning and health systems management. Numerous university-based health research units also contribute studies that are relevant to health decision-makers at the regional, provincial and federal levels.

5.   Physical and human resources

The non-financial inputs into the Canadian health system include physical, human and information technology resources. Although almost all such resources can be assigned a financial value, and are measured as such in terms of health expenditures in *section 4*, they should be analysed as inputs in their own right. The Commission on the Future of Health Care in Canada defined sustainability as the sufficiency of physical and human resources (and the funding necessary to mobilize these resource) – and their appropriate balance – to provide timely access to quality health services (Canada 2002). In addition, these services should be constantly adjusted in order to address the changing health needs of the population.

5.1   Physical resources

Provincial, territorial and federal ministries of health plan for the investment in – as well as the distribution of – infrastructure for public health care. Some of the decision-making on infrastructure is delegated by provincial ministries to regional health authorities, although most major investment decisions will be made in conjunction with the appropriate ministry since health ministers are ultimately accountable for the long-range planning of the overall health system within their respective jurisdictions.

5.1.1   Infrastructure and capital investment

Based on forecast data for 2004, C$5.9 billion was spent in Canada on construction, machinery and major equipment in the health sector, a capital investment that constitutes approximately 4.5% of total health spending. Of this total outlay, approximately C$1.4 billion – or roughly 25% – was spent on private sector facilities and equipment including long-term residential facilities (nursing homes) and private diagnostic clinics (CIHI 2004f).

During the immediate post-war years, Canada experienced rapid growth in the number and size of hospitals due to the growth in demand for inpatient care. This construction boom was fuelled by national hospital construction grants provided to the provinces by the federal government and by the introduction of hospitalization in the first decades following the Second World War. By the mid-1960s, the investment in health capital had slowed, and by the 1980s and 1990s, provincial governments were encouraging hospital consolidation as well as a reduction in the number of small and inefficient hospitals (Mackenzie 2004).

As is the case with other OECD countries, Canada has experienced a decline in the number of hospitals. From the mid-1980s until the mid-1990s, there was a 20% drop in the total number of hospitals offering inpatient care, as provinces, regional health authorities and hospital boards closed, consolidated and converted existing establishments in an effort to reduce operating costs and increase organizational efficiencies (Tully and Saint-Pierre 1997).

The number of hospital beds in Canada peaked by the late 1960s and has been declining ever since (Fig. 5.1). More importantly there has been a deep and systematic decline in hospital admissions in the recent past (Table 5.1).

Fig. 5.1   Beds in acute care hospitals, 1980–2001

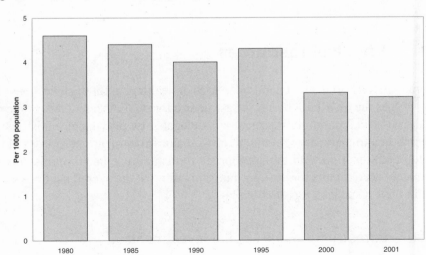

Source: OECD 2004a.

Table 5.1   Decline in the number of recorded hospital admissions for Canada and
provinces, 1995–2001

Province	% decline
British Columbia	-14.6
Alberta	-2.8
Saskatchewan	-19.2
Manitoba	-12.2
Ontario	-12.3
Quebec	-14.2
New Brunswick	-12.1
Nova Scotia	-19.1
Prince Edward Island	-12.8
Newfoundland and Labrador	-21.3
Canada	**-12.9**

Source: http://secure.cihi.ca/cihiweb/dispPage.jsp?cw_page=services_dad_e. CIHI discharge
abstract database, last updated 13 June 2005.

Note: The % decline is calculated on age-standardized hospitalization rates for all conditions,
per 100 000 population

Overall, the decline in hospital beds and the rate of hospitalization is due to
a number of factors, such as clinical practice changes – including the growth
in day (ambulatory) surgery as well as new surgical techniques – all pushed at
critical times by budgetary and capacity pressures (Barer et al. 2003; McGrail
et al. 2001; Evans et al. 2001). All provinces have experienced a decline in the
rate of hospital admissions (Table 5.1), though not necessarily in the average
time of hospital stay (Table 5.2). Based upon evidence from British Columbia,
the difference between the two results may be a consequence of that fact that
the data, as currently collected, includes long-term care patients in acute care
hospitals, thereby obscuring the real decline in acute care hospital stay (McGrail
et al. 2001).

Since almost all hospital care is considered an insured service under the
Canada Health Act, public funding is critical to decisions concerning capital
expansion and improvement. Public budgeting rules require that governments
and their delegates (including regional health authorities) carry capital
expenditures as current liabilities. As a consequence, there has been an incentive
to reduce capital expenditures more than operating expenditures during periods
of budgetary restraint. In addition, governments sometimes prefer not to
carry the burden of financing new hospital or other highly expensive health
infrastructure "up front".

As a consequence, some governments and regional health authorities have
begun to explore private finance initiatives (PFI) – known as public–private
partnerships or "P3s" in Canada. P3s allow governments to avoid potential

Table 5.2   Average length of hospital stay (in days) for Canada, provinces and
              territories, 1995, 2000 and 2001

Province	1995	2000	2001	% change: 2000–2001	% change: 1995–2001
British Columbia	6.4	7.1	7.2	1.4	12.5
Alberta	5.8	6.6	6.9	4.5	19.0
Saskatchewan	6.8	6.0	6.0	0.0	-11.8
Manitoba	9.3	9.5	9.2	-3.2	-1.1
Ontario	6.6	6.5	6.5	0.0	-1.5
Quebec	9.0	8.3	8.4	1.2	-6.7
New Brunswick	6.7	7.1	7.2	1.4	7.5
Nova Scotia	7.3	8.0	8.2	2.5	12.3
Prince Edward Island	7.6	8.1	8.1	0.0	6.6
Newfoundland/Labrador	7.6	7.8	7.7	-1.3	1.3
Yukon	4.0	5.1	5.2	2.0	30.0
Northwest Territories	4.1	4.5	4.4	-2.2	n/a
Nunavut	n/a	3.3	3.2	-3.0	n/a
Canada	7.2	7.2	7.3	1.4	1.4

Source: CIHI Discharge Abstract Database.

Note: Hospitalizations from Nunavut are reported separately from the Northwest Territories
beginning from 1999/2000.

capital costs in exchange for an annual rental fee, although the evidence from
the PFI experience in the United Kingdom is that such arrangements can,
and often do, cost the public purse more in the long run (Mackenzie 2004;
Sussex 2001).

In terms of new hospitals in Canada, P3s are largely at the planning and
construction stage including the William Osler and Royal Ottawa Hospitals in
Ontario. Private consortia have financed the construction of the building. Based
upon an inventory completed in April 2004, there were at least two P3 hospitals
in the final stages of construction: the Southland Health Centre, a C$400 million
multi-service diagnostic and treatment centre in Calgary; and the Academic
Ambulatory Care Centre, an outpatient clinic in Vancouver. In addition to
these imminent P3s, the Abbotsford hospital near Vancouver is expected to be
operational by 2007, and the Government of Quebec is considering two C$800
million P3 "super-hospitals" in Montreal (CUPE 2004).

5.1.2   Information technology

Based upon Statistics Canada's household Internet use survey for 2002, 62%
of all Canadian households had at least one member who used the Internet
regularly, over double the number in 1997. In addition, 52% of all Canadian

households had at least one member who regularly used the Internet from home. A majority of home Internet users accessed the Internet through a high-speed cable rather than a dial-up connection. While e-mailing and general browsing remain the two chief activities reported, the next most common activity was accessing the Internet for medical and health-related information. Almost two thirds of regular home Internet users relied upon the Internet to search for medical and health-related information in 2002, a major increase from the 43% that did so in 1998 (Statistics Canada *The Daily*, 18 September 2003). As noted in *sections 2.2* and *3.2*, health technology infrastructure has been established in the provinces, and supported by the Advisory Committee on Information and Emerging Technologies.

The word "telehealth" is used to describe a diverse array of developments from image transmission, telediagnostic services, telerobotic surgery to community-based applications such as teletriage and telehomecare. In 2004, Canada Health Infoway launched a strategy targeting investments in a series of telehealth applications in Aboriginal, official-language, minority, northern, rural and remote communities. To date, there have been few systematic studies of the impact of telehealth applications.

5.1.3   Medical equipment, devices and aids

Consistent with a decentralized public health care delivery system, Canada has a decentralized process of purchasing and procuring medical aids and devices. Although provincial ministries of health are ultimately responsible for their respective health systems, health organizations and providers actually purchase most medical aids and devices. At the same time, most physicians also maintain private offices and make independent decisions concerning the purchase of equipment from the basic diagnostic equipment, devices and aids in the general practitioner's office, for example, to ultrasounds in the paediatrician's office, to the numerous devices and medical equipment in an ophthalmologist's office.

In both regionalized and non-regionalized provinces, individual clinicians, particularly specialist physicians, also have a major role in the decision to purchase medical equipment, devices and aids, including at times the selection of the vendor if a particular piece of equipment or device has unique features associated with it. And in both regionalized and non-regionalized provinces, provincial health ministries play a key role in the timing and procurement of expensive medical equipment, particularly advanced diagnostic technology such as magnetic resonance imaging (MRI) units and computed tomography (CT) scanners. Table 5.3 shows the number of MRI units, CT and positron emission tomography (PET) scanners per million people from 1990 to 2004.

Table 5.3   Diagnostic imaging technologies (per million people), selected years

	1990	1995	2000	2004
Magnetic resonance imaging (MRI) units	0.7	1.3	2.5	4.8
Computed tomography (CT) scanners	7.1	8.0	9.5[a]	10.6
Positron emission tomography (PET) scanners	–	–	–	0.5

Source: CIHI 2004f.

Note: [a] 2001 data.

From the early to mid-1990s, provinces severely constrained their spending on health capital including advanced diagnostic equipment. This created a bottleneck in the system, increasing waiting times for numerous procedures and conditions (Canada 2002). Although public investment in advanced diagnostics has recently attempted to address this deficit, Canada's overall investment was low relative to all comparison countries and well below the OECD average as late as 1999. Recognizing the bottleneck, governments in Canada have focused on increasing the supply of equipment and supporting technical and professional personnel. As part of the 2000 first ministers' agreement on health, the federal government created a C$1 billion Medical Equipment Fund to assist provinces to purchase diagnostic and medical equipment in short supply (CICS 2000).

This initiative was extended in the 2003 first ministers' agreement through the creation of a C$1.5 billion Diagnostic/Medical Equipment Fund for both equipment – particularly advanced diagnostic equipment – and the training needed for specialized staff (CICS 2003). While these funds expire in the 2005/2006 fiscal year, the 2004 first ministers' agreement provided for an additional C$500 million investment in medical equipment (CICS 2004).

Table 5.4 displays the variation in the distribution of CT scanners and MRIs among the provinces and reflects the extent to which they have invested in advanced diagnostic equipment since 2000.

Most CT scanners and MRIs are funded by provincial and territorial governments as part of their commitment to provide diagnostic services as an insured service under the Canada Health Act. Most of this medical imaging equipment is located in hospitals, although as of 2004, 10 of the 286 CT scanners in the country were in free-standing facilities, while 20 MRIs, out of a total of 103, were in free-standing clinics. Most of the free-standing facilities are private-for-profit clinics that obtain the bulk of their funding from private sources including out-of-pocket payments and private insurance, as well as a small amount of public revenue through workers' compensation board payments, although some also obtain revenues from provincial governments for servicing Medicare patients for a set number of hours per week (CIHI 2004f). The emergence of private advanced diagnostic clinics has sparked a debate as

Fig. 5.2   **Selected imaging technologies (per million people), Canada and selected countries, latest available year**

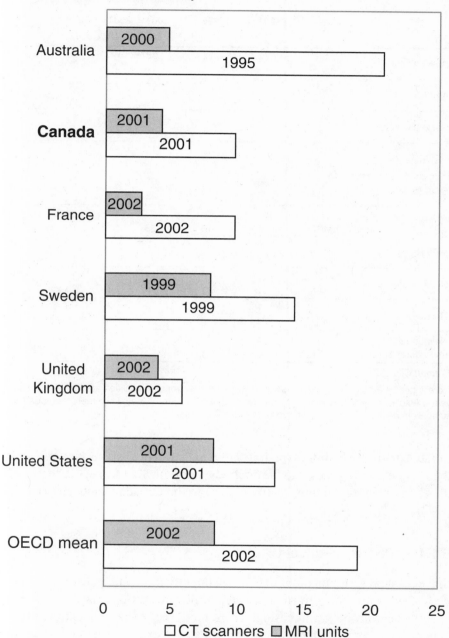

Source: OECD 2004a, CIHI 2004a.

Note: CT and MRI units located in hospitals and free-standing clinics but not in private sector facilities.

Table 5.4 Provincial distribution of CT Scanners and MRIs, 1991–2003

		1991	1995	2001	2003	2004	Rate per million people (2004)
British Columbia	CT	23	25	38	44	44	10.5
	MRI	3	7	14	18	19	4.5
Alberta	CT	22	23	25	30	30	9.3
	MRI	2	6	23	23	23	7.2
Saskatchewan	CT	5	6	9	10	11	11.1
	MRI	1	1	3	3	3	3.0
Manitoba	CT	8	10	13	14	17	14.2
	MRI	1	1	3	3	3	2.6
Ontario	CT	65	79	91	95	99	8.0
	MRI	10	12	44	49	52	4.2
Quebec	CT	58	68	92	94	98	13.0
	MRI	4	10	35	38	40	5.3
New Brunswick	CT	6	7	9	9	9	12.0
	MRI	0	1	5	5	5	6.7
Nova Scotia	CT	7	9	14	15	15	16.0
	MRI	1	1	2	4	4	4.3
Prince Edward Island	CT	1	1	2	2	3	21.8
	MRI	0	0	0	0	1	7.2
Newfoundland and Labrador	CT	5	6	9	10	10	19.3
	MRI	0	1	1	1	1	1.9

Source: CIHI 2004b.

Note: Units located both in hospitals and in free-standing imaging facilities are included for all years. As of 2004, there were no MRI scanners in the three territories while there was one CT scanner in each of the Yukon and the Northwest Territories.

to the extent to which they permit individuals to purchase faster service and then to queue-jump back into the public system with their respective test results thus contravening the universality criteria in the Canada Health Act (Canada 2002).

5.1.4 Pharmaceuticals

Since most prescription drugs are bought directly from pharmacists by patients with a prescription, governments and health institutions have had limited experience with bulk purchasing. There are three modest exceptions to this general rule. A few provincial governments have experimented with volume-discount agreements for new prescription drugs as a pre-condition to placement on their respective formularies. Following the terrorist attacks of 11 September 2001, the federal government attempted to prepare for a potential bio-terrorist attack by bulk-purchasing ciproflaxin, potassium iodide and smallpox vaccines. Finally, there have been examples of hospitals collaborating in the bulk purchase of drugs regularly used in acute care treatments (Yalnizyan 2004b).

The majority of pharmacists are salaried and work for private-for-profit commercial pharmacies. Depending upon the type of drug and the eligibility of the patient, a given prescription drug may be subsidized through private health insurance or public drug plans. (See *section 4.1.4* for a description of the regulation of the pharmaceutical sector.)

5.2   Human resources: trends, training, planning and registration/licensing

Family physicians continue to provide the majority of primary care services to Canadians. Most are engaged in private practice on a fee-for-service basis. Recently, some general practitioners have chosen to practise in multi-provider primary care teams as well as to accept blended forms of remuneration (see *section 3.5.2*). There is virtually no rostering of patients by family physicians and patients' choice of physicians is unencumbered in almost all cases.

Table 5.5   Health care personnel per 1000 people, 1991–2002

	1991	1995	2000	2001	2002
Family physicians	1.07	1.03	1.00	1.00	1.01
Specialist physicians	1.05	1.08	1.10	1.10	1.10
Registered nurses	–	7.93	7.58	7.46	7.36
Dentists	0.52	0.54	0.56	0.57	0.57
Pharmacists	0.71	0.76	0.80	0.83	0.84
Physiotherapists	0.39	0.43	0.47	0.47	0.48
Optometrists	0.10	0.10	0.11	0.11	0.11
Medical laboratory technicians	0.70	0.65	0.58	0.58	0.59
Medical radiation technologists	0.50	0.49	0.47	0.47	0.47
Occupational therapists	0.19	0.24	0.29	0.30	0.31
Psychologists	0.33	0.38	0.41	0.42	0.43
Chiropractors	0.14	0.15	0.18	0.20	0.20
Midwives	0.00	0.00	0.01	0.01	0.01

Sources: CIHI 2004b; Statistics Canada: CANSIM, Table 051–0001.

As seen in Table 5.5, by the early 1990s, specialist physicians had begun to outnumber family physicians, despite the fact that the training required to become a specialist was increased over this time period. Two factors account for this shift. The first is the increasing desire on the part of medical students to choose a specialization rather than family medicine. The second reason is that the family practice residence period was increased from one to two years, effectively eliminating an entire graduating cohort (Chan 2002a).

Physician specializations have increased dramatically with time. The Royal College of Physicians and Surgeons, which is responsible for overseeing the postgraduate training of physicians, now recognizes 60 specialist and sub-specialist areas of medical, surgical and laboratory medicine. The Royal College has 38 000 members. Specialists are certified by the Royal College, which is recognized by all provincial medical licensing authorities, except for Quebec, where the Collège des médecins du Québec is the primary certifying body. The total number of physician specialists has continued to grow (albeit gradually) throughout most of the 1990s and afterwards.

Fig. 5.3   Active physicians (per 1000 population), 1980–latest available year, Canada and selected countries

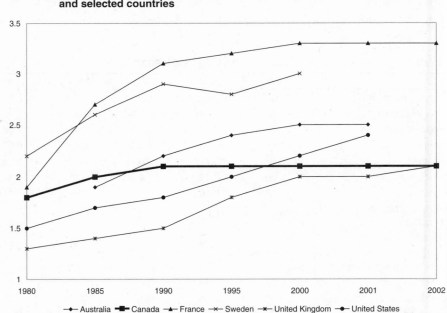

Source: OECD 2004a.

Canada along with the United Kingdom has fewer physicians per 1000 population than other comparison countries. More importantly, the rate of growth in the number of physicians in Canada has been slower than the five comparison countries from 1980 to the present. In addition, some jurisdictions such as Saskatchewan and Newfoundland and Labrador are highly dependent on hiring international medical graduates (see Table 5.6).

Table 5.6   Distribution of international medical graduates, by province, 2003

Province/territory	Total physicians per 1 000	Canadian MD graduates	International MD graduates	% distribution of international MD graduates
British Columbia	2.0	6038	2308	27.7
Alberta	1.83	4242	1492	31.8
Saskatchewan	1.53	721	797	52.5
Manitoba	1.77	1337	573	30.0
Ontario	1.77	16 541	5187	23.9
Quebec	2.07	13 788	1711	11.0
New Brunswick	1.63	952	269	22.0
Nova Scotia	2.09	1427	524	26.9
Prince Edward Island	1.41	159	29	15.4
Newfoundland/Labrador	1.88	552	372	40.3
Yukon	1.75	33	11	31.3
Northwest Territories	1.02	35	8	14.6
Nunavut	0.34	7	4	30.0
Canada	**1.87**	**45 832**	**13 407**	**22.5**

Source: CIHI 2004e.

Note: Total physicians include family/general practitioners, specialists, residents and interns. Canadian and foreign graduates exclude residents. Numbers may not total due to the exclusion of "unknown place of graduation". The small discrepancy between this table and Figure 5.3 is due to CIHI and OECD data differences.

Nurses outnumber all other health care personnel in the Canadian health system. Nurses can be classified in two broad groupings: regulated nurses including registered nurses, nurse practitioners, registered/licensed practical nurses and psychiatric nurses; and unregulated nurses including nurses' aides and orderlies. The description that follows focuses on the regulated nursing professions.

Registered nurses outnumber physicians, both family practitioners and specialists, by a factor of almost four. Among the nursing professions, registered nurses (RNs) constitute the largest sub-group, while licensed/registered practical nurses (LPNs) are the second largest group. During the 1990s, the number of

RNs declined by 8% and the number of LPNs declined by 21% (Canada 2002). These declines were a product of government cutbacks in the early to mid-1990s combined with an increase in nursing qualifications (CIHI 2004b).

Nurse practitioners, defined as registered nurses whose extra training and education entitles them to an "extended class" designation, are currently on the front line of health reform, particularly primary care reform. Their scope of practice – which includes prescribing some prescription drug therapies and ordering some diagnostic tests – overlaps with the scope of practice of general practitioners/family physicians. More importantly, given the evidence of the "declining comprehensiveness" of the primary care offered by physicians since the late 1980s, the range of health services offered by nurse practitioners should be of great interest in future primary health reforms (Chan 2002b; Ontario 2005; College of Nurses of Ontario 2004).

Fig. 5.4   Active nurses per 1000 in Canada and selected countries, 1980–2002

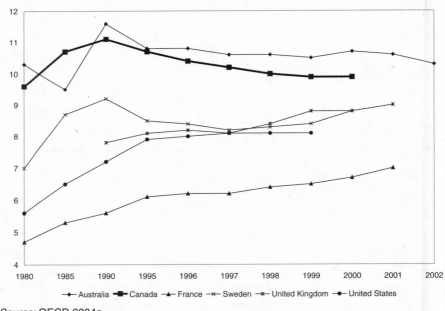

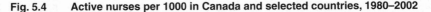

Source: OECD 2004a.

Relative to the group of comparison countries, Canada is second only to Australia in terms of the per capita number of nurses. At the same time, Canada's decline in the per capita number of nurses in the 1990s is unmatched by any other country. On the contrary, over this same period, France, the United Kingdom and the United States have experienced a substantial increase in their per capita number of nurses. However, some caution should be applied to these comparisons given potential differences among countries in their respective definitions of nurses.

Along with the increase in the use of prescription drugs, pharmacists are growing in number in Canada. There are over 26 300 licensed pharmacists in Canada. Most pharmacists are employed by commercial pharmacies (about 72%), dispensing drugs to individuals who have received prescriptions from doctors. About 15% of pharmacists are employed by hospitals to dispense drugs needed by patients receiving acute care, and an even smaller number are part of health provider teams. Training consists of a Bachelor's degree in pharmacy from a Canadian university, a national board examination and practical experience through internship. The Canadian Pharmacists Association, a national voluntary organization, represents the interests of pharmacists in Canada.

Medical laboratory technologists and medical radiation technologists are essential in supporting many of the diagnostic and treatment tools used by physicians. While both groups were affected by the government cutbacks in the early to mid-1990s, their numbers have begun to grow with increased public investment in health in the late 1990s. Both groups of technologists are certified by national organizations – the Canadian Society for Medical Laboratory Science and the Canadian Association for Medical Radiation Technologists – but they are self-regulated at the provincial level. Education and training vary from two to five years depending on the designation and degree of specialization. Medical radiation technologists specialize in one of four areas: radiography, radiation therapy, nuclear medicine and magnetic resonance imaging.

The number of dentists per 1000 population has grown steadily since 1991 (see Table 5.5). Since most of these services are delivered outside the public health care system, the number of dentists has not been influenced, positively or negatively, by the sharp fluctuations in public investment. Among OECD countries, Canada has the fourth highest rate of total per capita dental expenditures but the second lowest public per capita public dental expenditures (Baldota and Leake 2004). This simply reflects the fact that most dental care in Canada is funded, administered and delivered privately.

As with physicians, a number of specializations requiring additional postsecondary education and residency requirements have emerged over time including (but not limited to): orthodontists, periodontists, endodontists and paediatric dentists. A four-year university programme is required for general dentistry, while another two to three years of postgraduate residency is required for specialization.

A number of allied dental professionals support dentists and dental specialists in their work, including dental assistants and dental hygienists. Provincial dental organizations are responsible for licensing and self-regulating various professional sub-groups, although the Royal College of Dentists of Canada plays a similar role to the Royal College of Physicians and Surgeons of Canada in setting standards for postgraduate education and training.

Physiotherapists, occupational therapists, psychologists and chiropractors have all seen a dramatic increase in demand for their health care services since the early 1990s. All are self-governing professions with provincial licensing and regulatory frameworks that vary, sometimes considerably, from jurisdiction to jurisdiction.

To practise, physiotherapists must graduate from an accredited university physiotherapy programme and meet all provincial or territorial licensing requirements. A growing number are now assisted by rehabilitation assistants. In addition, British Columbia, Alberta, Ontario, Prince Edward Island, Nova Scotia and Newfoundland and Labrador require applicants to pass a national physiotherapy competency exam. The profession has recently issued a strategic review recommending national health human resource planning for the longer term (Canadian Alliance of Physiotherapy Regulators and the Canadian Physiotherapy Association 2002).

Although occupational therapists are currently required to have an undergraduate degree from an accredited university programme, the profession will require a professional Master's degree by the end of the decade (Canadian Association of Occupational Therapists, 2002). Occupational therapists can be distinguished from physiotherapists in providing advice on the workplace. As is the case with other health care professions, occupational therapists are increasing educational and training requirements in order to protect and expand their scope of practice.

The growing demand for psychological services has largely been funded privately, outside provincial and territorial public health care plans. Despite mounting evidence concerning the efficacy of numerous psychological treatments, and the major challenge of mental health, governments have been reluctant to extend public coverage to psychological therapies (Romanow and Marchildon 2003). Provinces vary in terms of licensing requirements, but most require graduation from an accredited graduate university programme in order to practice as a psychologist.

Chiropractors require four to five years of postsecondary education plus another two to three years of internship. Provincially self-regulated, chiropractic scope of practice varies from jurisdiction to jurisdiction but only a few provincial health plans (Alberta, Saskatchewan and Manitoba) cover selected chiropractic services. In contrast, chiropractic treatment is covered quite extensively under private health insurance plans. There are two accredited chiropractic programmes in Canada: the Canadian Memorial Chiropractic College in Toronto and the Université de Québec à Trois-Rivières.

Optometrists must complete a four-year doctor of optometry programme as well as meet provincial licensing requirements to practise. Entry into such programmes is dependent upon some undergraduate education in mathematics or science. There are two accredited optometry programmes in Canada: the University of Waterloo with 240 students, and the Université de Montréal with 160 students. Optometrists are supported in their work by optometric assistants.

In 1994, Ontario was the first province to establish regulation of midwives, to fund midwifery services as part of the public system and to provide an undergraduate university programme. Currently, midwifery is also being integrated into the public health care systems of British Columbia, Alberta, Manitoba and Quebec while Saskatchewan and Nova Scotia have announced their intention to do so as well. While a local system of midwifery was prevalent in Canada in the 19th century, it had virtually disappeared until being "reborn" in the mid- to late 1970s as part of the women's movement and the counterculture's "home birth movement". By the 1990s, a pronounced trend towards professionalization of midwifery had occurred, including professional self-regulation and standardized baccalaureate degree programmes (Bourgeault 2000).

With the increasing emphasis on illness prevention and health promotion by public health organizations and government ministries, dieticians, nutritionists and similar health advisers providers are becoming a more visible part of the health workforce. In addition, with the expansion of community health centres in some provinces, public health practitioners, social workers, community outreach workers and advisers are also becoming more common.

These developments in "upstream" health combined with primary care reform place considerable emphasis on the ability of interdisciplinary teams to work effectively together. Although no dedicated research institute has been established in Canada to conduct applied research on inter-professional collaboration, Health Canada directs and funds an initiative in interdisciplinary education for collaborative patient-centred care.

6.   Provision of services

6.1   Public health

Public health is often defined as the science and art of promoting health, preventing disease, and prolonging life through the organized efforts of society. In Canada, public health is generally identified with the following six discrete functions: population health assessment; health promotion; disease and injury control and prevention; health protection; surveillance; and emergency preparedness and response. In all cases, public health policies and programmes are focused on the population as a whole in contrast to health care policies and programmes that tend to be focused on the individual.

The federal, provincial and territorial governments, as well as regional health authorities, perform some or all of these functions, and all governments appoint a chief public/medical health officer to lead their public health efforts in their respective jurisdictions. These individuals are generally physicians with a specialized training and education in public health. By virtue of their extensive responsibilities for health care, provincial ministries of health all have public health branches covering virtually all public health issues. In addition, some provinces have initiated major population health initiatives in recent years.

The federal government provides a broad range of public health services through various means, although the recently established Public Health Agency of Canada has the mandate to provide or coordinate the six public health functions mentioned above. With its partners in the voluntary sector, the Public Health Agency of Canada is responsible for a number of health promotion and illness prevention activities including the Aboriginal Head Start Program, the Canada Prenatal Nutrition Program and the Healthy Living Strategy.

Through federal/provincial agreement, national initiatives aimed at reducing child poverty and increasing the health of children were launched in the 1990s. The programmes and initiatives surrounding the Children's Action Plan and the National Child Benefit are administered by a number of ministries joined by a myriad of voluntary organizations.

6.1.1 Health promotion, illness prevention and public health education

As part of their respective public health care plans, the provinces and territories have established public health promotion and education as well as illness prevention initiatives. In addition, because of their explicit population health mandates, regional health authorities have initiated their own public health promotion and education, and illness prevention programmes have focused on the areas of greatest need.

The federal government also runs a number of health promotion and education programmes concerning alcohol and drug abuse, family violence, fetal alcohol syndrome, food and nutrition, mental health, physical activity, safety and injury, and sexuality, including AIDS prevention. This list also includes tobacco reduction, and the Health Canada's Tobacco Control Strategy has been one of the more ambitious national programmes among OECD countries. In conjunction with a large number of Canadian organizations, Health Canada has also spearheaded one of the most comprehensive e-health information websites in the world providing reliable information for all Canadians on how to stay healthy and prevent illness.

In 2002, in response to the growing obesity problem, the federal, provincial and territorial health ministers launched the Integrated Pan-Canadian Healthy Living Strategy. This intergovernmental plan attempts to improve the state of knowledge, as well as coordinate governmental and voluntary initiatives, concerned with encouraging physical activity and healthier eating.

Improved health promotion as well as enhanced disease and injury prevention are major elements in any effective system of primary health care. As such, they are expected to become key components of the primary care reforms currently being initiated in the provinces and territories (see *section 6.3*).

The Canadian Public Health Association (CPHA) is a voluntary organization dedicated to improving the state of public health in Canada. The CPHA, along with its provincial and territorial branches or associations, is heavily engaged in promoting public health education and illness prevention initiatives.

6.1.2   Screening programmes

The provincial and territorial ministries of health have implemented screening programmes for early detection of cancer that vary considerably in approach, delivery and comprehensiveness. Since the 1970s, considerable intergovernmental effort has gone into creating a pan-Canadian strategy for cancer screening. By the 1990s, national screening initiatives in breast and cervical cancer had been launched. An informal association of federal and provincial representatives in conjunction with the relevant clinical professions, the Cervical Cancer Prevention Network, was established to work on three aspects of a provincially based but national screening programme in 1995 (Health Canada 1998):

• effective patient recruitment strategies;

• required information systems to support comprehensive screening;

• quality practice guidelines to support provincially managed screening programmes.

With funding from Health Canada, the Canada Breast Cancer Screening Initiative, with a twin focus on public education and programme development, was also launched in the 1990s. Through this initiative a national screening database was established, derived from provincial breast screening data.

Provincial efforts at comprehensive screening vary considerably. Through Cancer Care Ontario, the province of Ontario has been a leader in providing comprehensive breast screening services. Approximately 100 centres scattered throughout the province have been approved by the Ontario Breast Screening Program to provide a service for women aged 50 and over. Provinces such as British Columbia and Saskatchewan also have comprehensive breast screening programmes.

In 2003, the Government of Ontario established the first major colorectal cancer screening pilot programme in the country. By way of contrast, there has been no major intergovernmental screening initiative on colorectal cancer – a relatively treatable cancer that is second only to lung cancer in Canada in terms of mortality.

6.1.3   Communicable disease control

All provincial and territorial ministries of health devote resources to communicable disease control within their jurisdictions. But given the geographical reach of communicable diseases and the rapidity with which they spread, the federal government has often been called upon to play a larger role in controlling communicable diseases. The SARS outbreak in 2003 and the

Naylor report that followed in its wake were the catalysts for a policy change many considered overdue (Health Canada 2003a). In response to the report, the federal government expanded its national infectious disease control and prevention infrastructure (comparable in at least some respects to the Centers for Disease Control and Prevention in the United States).

Established in 2004, the Public Health Agency of Canada was given a mandate to prepare for, and respond to, infectious disease epidemics, including emergency preparedness. The Public Health Agency's office in Winnipeg, Manitoba, has also become the home for the newly created International Centre for Infectious Diseases (ICID), a multi-sector partnership (federal, provincial, and municipal governments along with private industry) that fosters collaboration between scientists and infectious disease professionals. ICID has a mandate to encourage economic development around the commercialization of research in public health.

6.1.4   Immunization

Provincial and territorial ministries of health are primarily responsible for immunization planning and programmes. Actual immunization can be delivered in a number of ways but the two most common are through regional public health offices and family physicians. As shown in Table 1.6, in 1998 the rate of measles vaccination was 96.2%, while the rate of DPT vaccination was only 84.2% of children over 2 years old.

In 2004, the federal government launched a three-year C$400 million initiative targeting five preventable children's illnesses. This money will be transferred to the provinces and territories in order to purchase vaccines (C$300 million) and to support front-line delivery of public health services including vaccines (C$100 million).

6.2   Patient pathways

The decentralized nature of health delivery means that patient pathways do vary considerably across Canada, therefore the following steps are part of a highly stylized pathway of a woman named Mary living in the more southern and urban part of the country.

- Upon getting ill, Mary visits her family physician where she is given a preliminary examination. She is not permitted to seek out a specialist on her own.

- Depending on the diagnosis, Mary could be given a prescription for a drug therapy, a referral for further tests including a blood analysis or X-ray, or a referral to a specialist.

- If sent for further tests, Mary's results will be returned to the family physician. Once the physician receives the results, she will call Mary back to her office for a further consultation and, if necessary, explanation of the next steps in treatment.

- If referred to a specialist, Mary will be examined and a decision will be made concerning specialized treatment. Her family physician will be informed of the results of the specialist's diagnosis.

- If the treatment involves a surgical procedure or other acute intervention, Mary will be given a date to attend the hospital.

- While waiting for surgery, her specialist will prescribe any necessary medication for which Mary may pay or contribute towards, depending on whether she has private health insurance or is eligible for subsidy through her provincial or territorial drug plan. In contrast, her physician visits and hospital stay are considered to be medically necessary services and are free of charge to Mary.

- Upon Mary's discharge from the hospital, her family physician receives a discharge summary from her specialist and may check on Mary's progress some time later.

- If Mary requires home care or rehabilitation services in an outpatient centre, she may pay some of the costs. The amount Mary pays for these services will depend on the benefits offered in her province of residence.

6.3   Primary/ambulatory care

Primary health care can be defined as the first point of contact between an individual and the health system and, at its core, involves general medical care for common conditions and injuries. It can, and should, involve some of the health promotion and disease prevention activities already canvassed above under the heading of public health. General ambulatory care simply refers to non-acute medical services that are provided to an individual who arrives and leaves under his/her own locomotion.

In recent years, primary care has once again become the focus of public health care reform efforts in Canada. In September 2000, the first ministers of Canada's provinces, territories and central government agreed to work together on a comprehensive primary health care agenda, based on the following statement: "Improvements to primary care are crucial to the renewal of health services. Governments are committed to ensuring that Canadians receive the most appropriate care, by the most appropriate providers, in the most appropriate settings" (CICS 2000). The results of the consultations and the citizens' dialogue conducted by the Romanow Commission indicate that the desire for primary care change is also supported by the general public (Canada 2002; Maxwell et al. 2002). Finally, there is compelling evidence that supports the proposition that, for any defined population, more effective primary health care translates into improved health outcomes (Starfield 2004).

The traditional model of primary care in Canada has been one in which a family physician, working individually on a fee-for-service basis, provides general medical services to his/her patients. While rostering is not involved, most family physicians have a relatively stable group of patients after the initial period required to build up a medical practice. And while patients have freedom of choice in selecting a family physician, most choose to have long-standing relationships with their family physicians. However, the family physician's range of skills, as well as the impact of a volume-driven incentive system through fee-for-service payments, limits both diagnosis and treatment.

As a consequence, provinces and territories established a number of initiatives to improve primary care in the 1970s and 1980s. Working through primary care providers with a broader conception of their role (for instance, CLSC salaried physicians in Quebec) or through community clinics offering the services of other health professions in addition to family physicians, provinces and territories attempted to change their respective health systems. Even with all these innovations, however, there was only limited change by the end of the 1990s (Hutchison, Abelson and Lavis 2001). Fig. 6.1 illustrates the extent to which first contact with the health system for most Canadians is with a physician.

Since 2000, provinces and territories have renewed their efforts, in part as a consequence of the recent spate of health system reports that have placed primary health care at the very centre of the reform project, and change has become more evident. An inventory of provincial and territorial primary care reforms conducted at the end of 2003 highlights some of these changes. One of the potentially most significant steps is that a majority of provinces are changing their laws to enable nurse practitioners to deliver a broad range of primary care services. Another change is the willingness of some provinces, backed up by transfers from Ottawa, to make some major investments in primary health service organizations as well as in information infrastructure to accelerate the reforms. This is being accompanied by some jurisdictions setting targets concerning the replacement of fee-for-service remuneration by alternative payment contracts for physicians, by full-time (24/7) access to essential services

Fig. 6.1   Percentage of the population reporting outpatient contacts, 1994–2003

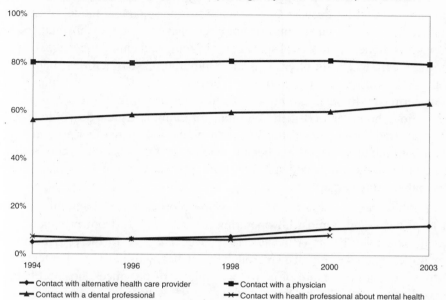

Source: Statistics Canada: CANSIM Tables 105–0260, 105–0261, 105–0262, 105–0263.

Notes: Population aged 12 and over who have reported contact in the past 12 months. Medical doctors include family or general practitioners as well as specialists such as surgeons, allergists, orthopaedists, gynaecologists, or psychiatrists. For population aged 18 and under, includes paediatricians. Dental professionals include dentists, orthodontists or dental hygienists. Alternative health care providers include: massage therapists, acupuncturists, homeopaths or naturopaths, Feldenkrais or Alexander teachers, relaxation therapists, biofeedback teachers, rolfers, herbalists, reflexologists, spiritual healers, religious healers, and others. Mental health professionals include: family doctors or general practitioners, psychiatrists, psychologists, nurses, social workers and counsellors.

and by accelerating the development of telehealth applications in rural, remote and northern areas of the country (Wilson, Shortt and Dorland 2004).

6.4   Secondary/inpatient and specialized ambulatory care

In Canada, virtually all secondary, tertiary and emergency care, as well as the majority of specialized ambulatory care and elective surgery, is performed within hospitals. While hospitals have traditionally been the centre of the Canadian health care universe, much health care reform has attempted to shift this emphasis to primary care, illness prevention and health promotion (Decter 2000).

Based upon the typology introduced by Healy and McKee (2002), the prevailing trend for decades has been toward the separatist model of hospital rather than the dominant, hub or comprehensive models of hospital. In the separatist model, the hospital specializes in acute and emergency care, leaving primary care to family physicians or community-based facilities such as the CLSCs in Quebec and the community health centres (CHCs) in Ontario, and long-term care to nursing homes and similar institutions. There are important exceptions, however. In British Columbia, for example, a great deal of long-term care has traditionally been attached to hospitals. There are other exceptions as well but the current trend has been to encourage the consolidation of tertiary care in fewer hospitals and spin off some types of elective surgery to highly specialized day surgery clinics.

For historical reasons, hospitals have been organized and administered on a local basis with almost all operating at arm's length from provincial and territorial governments (Boychuk 1999; Deber 2004). In the provinces and territories that have embraced regionalization, hospitals have been "integrated" into a broader continuum of care. In a number of provinces, hospital boards have been dismantled in favour of larger RHA boards, except in Ontario where hospital boards exercise considerable influence within the provincial community.

Recently, the Ontario Hospital Association and the Government of Ontario in association with the University of Toronto and the Canadian Institute for Health Information have conducted annual evaluations of acute care performance in all Ontario hospitals based upon a "balanced scorecard" approach (CIHI 2003c). The performance measures relied upon in these evaluations fall into four broad quadrants:

- system integration and change
- clinical utilization and outcomes
- patient satisfaction
- financial performance and condition.

These studies illustrate how hospitals, at least in Ontario, allocate resources. In 2001/2002, for example, 46% of total hospital expenditures was devoted to nursing services, 21% to diagnostic and therapeutic expenses (not including physicians), 24.7% to administration, and a final 7.2% to research, education, community services and reserves. From 1999/2000 to 2001/2002, same-day surgery volumes and ambulatory visits have each increased by more than 6%, while emergency centre visits increased by more than 3%. At the same time, inpatient admissions decreased by just over 1% (CIHI 2003c).

6.5   Pharmaceutical care

There are two basic reasons why family physicians retain the principal responsibility for primary care in Canada. First, despite some reform efforts to enlarge the professional primary care team, most primary care continues to be delivered by family physicians. Second, only physicians are legally permitted to prescribe a full range of pharmaceutical therapies (see *section 4.1.4* for more information on the regulation of the pharmaceutical sector). Within their scope of practice, dentists are permitted to use a limited range of prescription drugs. In some provinces and within their scope of practice, nurse practitioners are now permitted to prescribe a limited number of drugs.

After hospital care, prescription drug therapy combined with over-the-counter drugs (OTC) now constitutes the second largest category of health care expenditure in Canada, larger even than outlays for physician care. Over-the-counter drug spending has been relatively static compared to the growth in prescription drug expenditure which has, in turn, been fuelled by the introduction of new drugs and, to a lesser extent, by the increased use of older drugs.

Based upon a study using 2001 data, the average Canadian family of three accounted for over C$1200 a year in expenditure on prescription drugs with each member of the family obtaining 10 prescriptions a year at an average prescription price of almost C$40 (IMS HEALTH Canada et al. 2002).

The following is a list of the top ten therapeutic categories ranked by the number of prescriptions dispensed by Canadian retail pharmacies in 2003. The percentage of change over 2002 is indicated in brackets (IMS HEALTH Canada 2004):

- cardiovasculars (7.9%)
- psychotherapeutics (10.4%)
- hormones, including sex hormones (–6.7%)
- anti-infectives systemic (1.7%)
- analgesics (5.2%)
- antispasmodics/antisecretory (11.1%)
- cholesterol agents (17.7%)
- anti-arthritics (2.8%)
- bronchial therapy (2.7%)
- diuretics (11.8%).

While there are a large number of pharmacies scattered throughout Canada, most are part of chain stores, while a smaller number are independent pharmacies. Almost all pharmacies, whether they are independent or part of a chain, sell a host of products beyond prescription and OTC drugs. Large chain grocery stores now compete directly with the pharmacies by selling both prescription and OTC drugs. In 2003, there were 4447 outlets belonging to chain stores, 1616 outlets that were independent pharmacies, and 1396 outlets that were run by mass retailers, largely grocery stores (IMS HEALTH Canada 2004). Although regulated, the prescription drug sector in Canada is highly competitive at the retail level.

Pharmaceuticals are manufactured in Canada by resident firms as well as by the branch companies of international manufacturers. Despite a patent drug manufacturing sector concentrated in Quebec and a generic drug manufacturing industry concentrated in Ontario, Canada has always been reliant on the world market for a portion of its prescription drug needs, and recent trends suggest that it is becoming even less self-sufficient (Reichert and Windover 2002). In addition, the research and development-to-sales ratio has been declining steadily since 1998 (PMPRB 2004).

6.6   Rehabilitation/intermediate care

Rehabilitation can occur within or outside hospitals. Inpatient rehabilitation focuses on a number of conditions. Based upon a recent CIHI (2004) study, the five largest client groups, listed in descending order of frequency are: orthopaedics (mostly knee and hip replacements); stroke; brain dysfunction; amputation of limb; and spinal cord injury. Based upon the sample studied, the average age of an inpatient rehabilitation client was 70 years of age. The median length of stay varied from 13 days for arthritis patients to 44 days for patients with spinal cord injury, with an overall median length of stay of 22 days (CIHI 2004c).

Outpatient rehabilitation generally occurs in physiotherapy clinics. Depending on the provincial/territorial health plan or workers' compensation benefits, or the benefits conferred through (largely) employment-based private health insurance policies, some home care physiotherapy and workplace occupational therapy may also be made available, although all of these services can also be purchased out-of-pocket by those able to afford them.

6.7   Long-term care, home care and other community care

Community care services are organized according to the degree of care required and the location of that care. Community care outside the home is provided in institutions ranging from residential care facilities, which provide a range of limited assisted-living services, to chronic care facilities, which provide services to very high-need patients who may be suffering severe physical and mental disabilities. For individuals requiring less intensive care or living assistance, home-based care may be available, although its availability and quality varies considerably from province to province. In recent years, the private-for-profit home-care services have become more prevalent.

Most long-term care for the dependent, and often frail, elderly is provided in nursing homes. In the provinces that have undergone regionalization, some of these are run directly by the RHAs but a large number remain independent enterprises, often in a contractual relationship with the RHA to provide a given level of long-term care. There is also an active private-for-profit nursing home sector providing various levels of care to the elderly. Based upon a study analysing 1998/1999 fiscal data, expenditures for home care were estimated to be between C$2 and C$3 billion, while expenditures on long-term facilities were estimated to be C$7 billion compared to C$26 billion spent on hospitals (Ballinger et al. 2001).

Private not-for-profit as well as private-for-profit home and community care services are available throughout Canada. Similar public services are also available, although the terms and conditions vary considerably depending on the province or territory. As a general rule, long-term care services are paid for by the provincial or territorial government but accommodation and meal costs are the responsibility of the individual, unless means-testing demonstrates that the individual cannot afford such expenses.

6.8   Services for informal caregivers

Each province and territory has its own policies and programmes concerning support and services for informal caregivers. In most provinces and territories, these services are directly related to the package of public home care services offered by the relevant ministry of health.

Since 2002, the federal government has provided tax credits for eligible caregivers. Shortly afterwards, the federal government also introduced a change to the rules surrounding unemployment insurance, allowing employees the right to take a paid absence from work in order to provide home or end-of-life (palliative) care in defined circumstances. The 2004 federal budget changed the existing medical expense tax credit to allow caregivers to claim more than had been allowable in order to assist in the caring of children and dependent relatives. The compassionate family care benefit (through the federal Employment

Insurance Program) was introduced in 2004 to support those who need to leave their job temporarily to care for a gravely ill or dying child, parent, or spouse (Finance Canada 2004).

6.9   Palliative care

Modern palliative care practices in Canada can be traced back to the 1970s. These hospice palliative care programmes were developed by various community-based organizations in response to the needs of the dying. Today, there are over 600 such programmes across Canada although they vary considerably in terms of content. There is also considerable variability in terms of the access by Canadians to these services. The Canadian Hospice Palliative Care Association (Ferris et al. 2002) estimated that only a minority of Canadians facing a life-threatening illness had access to such programmes.

There is no national policy on palliative care in Canada. Instead, there are national guidelines developed by community-based palliative care organizations operating at arm's length from government. While the degree of variability in palliative care prompted the federal government to publish service guidelines in 1981, these were filled out by palliative care NGOs. In 1989, the Metropolitan Toronto Palliative Care Council and the British Columbia Hospice/Palliative Care Association worked together to develop more specific standards of palliative care practice and were joined two years later by the Ontario Palliative Care Association. By 1993, this work was being consolidated by the national umbrella organization. This work, achieved through consensus with all the major community-based palliative organizations, finally culminated in a standardized approach to hospice palliative care that is now becoming the national standard of care (Ferris et al. 2002).

In the late 1990s, a Senate Committee under Senator Sharon Carstairs conducted a review of palliative care, building upon the work of an earlier Special Senate Committee on Euthanasia and Assisted Suicide. Senator Carstairs' committee's report – *Quality End-of-Life Care: The Right of all Canadians* – contained a number of recommendations to improve the state of knowledge concerning palliative care that could be the foundation upon which palliative care would be improved throughout Canada (Senate 2000). Since this report, a Secretariat on Palliative and End-of-Life Care was established within Health Canada. This secretariat is currently working with the Canadian Council on Health Services Accreditation to develop and implement standards and indicators for palliative programmes and services.

6.10   Mental health care

Over the past half-century, mental health care has moved from predominantly institutional care to ambulatory and community care as a consequence of changing professional therapies in conjunction with the introduction of new prescription drug therapies. Canada has followed the same "deinstitutionalization trend" as other wealthy OECD countries. For historical reasons, however, some mental health care services have never been fully incorporated within the universal portion of the public health system. Psychological services, for example, are not considered "insured services" under the terms of the Canada Health Act largely because they are non-physician outpatient services (Romanow and Marchildon 2003).

Mental disorders and diseases appear to be growing throughout the OECD, yet all countries, including Canada, are not adequately addressing this challenge through new public health care approaches and infrastructure (WHO 2001). The result is shown in Table 1.4 where deaths from mental and behavioural disorders have increased quite dramatically between 1970 and the 2001.

6.11   Dental health care

Almost all dental health services are delivered by independent dental practitioners operating their own businesses. Payment for these services is through private health insurance or direct out-of-pocket payment. If a provincial or territorial resident is receiving social assistance, then a portion or all of the costs for dental services may be covered.

Approximately 94% of all dentistry is provided outside the public system. Although dental fees are not regulated, prices are generally in line with private insurance payout guidelines. Private health insurance is responsible for slightly more than 50% of funding for dental services in Canada (Baldota and Leake 2004).

The exception to this largely private model is dental surgery performed in a hospital as an insured service, as defined under the Canada Health Act. Another exception concerns public dental service programmes for school children. The first provincial programme of this type was launched by the Government of Saskatchewan under the New Democratic Party in the 1970s. Utilizing dental nurses and paraprofessionals, the Saskatchewan Dental Program proved to be highly effective but was disbanded within a decade by a newly elected

Progressive Conservative government in Saskatchewan in the 1980s (Wolfson 1997). Some targeted dental programmes – such as the CINOT (children in need of treatment) programme in Ontario – are offered by a few provincial governments.

6.12 Complementary and alternative health products and services

Complementary and alternative medicine (CAM) embraces entire systems of medicine, such as traditional Chinese medicine and Aboriginal healing, as well as specific medicines and therapies such as herbalism, relaxation therapy and reflexology. Jonas and Levin (1999) have catalogued some 4000 different CAM practices including homeopathy, chiropractic and therapeutic massage. Although these practices vary considerably, most CAM therapies share at least four common characteristics (Health Canada 2003c):

- they are presumed to work in conjunction with the body's own self-healing mechanisms;
- they are "holistic" in the sense that they treat the whole person;
- they try to involve the individual "patient" as an active participant in the healing process;
- they focus on disease prevention and wellbeing as much as on treatment.

As is the case in most OECD countries, Canadians have shown increasing interest in CAM, and the rate of growth in the number of alternative practitioners is beginning to outstrip the rate of growth in mainstream health care providers (Clarke 2004; Sutherland and Verhoef 1994). At the same time, the response of the established health care professions to the emerging CAM practitioners ranges from scepticism to hostility (Kelner et al. 2004). Some CAM groups, including naturopaths, traditional Chinese medicine acupuncturists and homeopaths, have responded to these challenges by pursuing a strategy to professionalize (Welsh et al. 2004).

There are approximately 50 000–60 000 natural health products on the Canadian market. Of this number, approximately 10 000 natural health products have gone through a Health Canada approval process. In 2004, Health Canada established a Natural Health Products Directorate that is now responsible for regulating such products (see *section 4.1.3*).

6.13   Maternal and child health care

Maternal and child health services have not typically been addressed separately from other health services, except to the extent that professional specialization offers services specifically to mothers and their children. This specialization has occurred among physicians, dentists and psychologists to name but a few. The one exception is midwifery, an older health profession that was virtually extinguished following the Second World War and is only now beginning to make a comeback by following the model of professional accreditation and self-regulation common to most other organized health providers (Bourgeault 2000; Clarke 2004).

Most maternal and child health care is primary care, and the bulk of this continues to be provided by family physicians. While there are some important exceptions – pre- and postnatal maternal and infant programmes through community health centres, for example – maternal and child care has not been given separate emphasis by provincial ministries and regional health authorities. This is so despite the fact that single mothers in Canada have poor health status relative to countries such as Norway with a more targeted approach to maternal and child health care (Curtis and Phipps 2004). With the introduction of primary care teams involving other health providers, perhaps including child psychologists and midwives, more targeted services may be provided at this level in the future.

6.14   Health care and Aboriginal Canadians

Multiple indicators demonstrate that the health status of Aboriginal Canadians is well below the Canadian average. And while Aboriginal health status has improved in the post-war period, relative to overall Canadian health status, a significant gap continues to persist. As with Aboriginal populations in other OECD countries such as Australia, New Zealand and the United States, the reasons for this state of affairs have long historical roots (Waldram, Herring and Young 1995).

Historically, federal, provincial and territorial government efforts to meet the health needs of Aboriginal Canadians have achieved only limited success. As a consequence, Aboriginal organizations and leaders have argued for greater control over the funding and delivery of health services. In the last decade, a series of health funding transfer agreements between the federal government and eligible First Nations and Inuit organizations has permitted a degree of Aboriginal control, particularly in areas of primary health care (Lavoie 2004).

More than the transfer of control of existing health care delivery, this new Aboriginal health movement involves a different philosophy and approach to health and health care. According to Lemchuk-Favel and Jock (2004), the strengths of the Aboriginal health movement include self-empowerment, holistic healing that takes a culturally distinct approach to primary health care, including an emphasis on the synergies produced by combining indigenous healing and medicines with western health approaches. The challenges faced by the Aboriginal health movement include small community size, the remoteness of many Aboriginal populations, limited funding and the prevalence of diabetes and fetal alcohol syndrome within their communities.

7.   Principal health care reforms

7.1   Analysis of recent reforms

The purpose of this section is to review the Canadian health reform experience of the last 15 years. Of particular note is the linkage between the recommendations made in numerous arm's-length studies of provincial and national public health care systems and the reforms actually implemented by both orders of government working separately or, at times, collaboratively.

The modern era of Canadian health care reform began shortly after the passage of the Canada Health Act (1984). In one sense, this federal legislation locked in place a pattern of universal coverage that had originally been set up through the Hospital Insurance and Diagnostic Services Act (1957) and the Medical Care Act (1966). By withdrawing transfer funding from those jurisdictions permitting user fees and extra charges on a dollar-for-dollar basis, and then returning most of the nearly C$250 million originally withdrawn after provinces eliminated such fees, the federal government ensured the "narrow but deep" coverage aspect of Canadian Medicare. Just as important, the Canada Health Act incorporated the criteria of public administration, comprehensiveness, universality and portability from the older legislation, while adding a fifth new principle – accessibility. This last principle states that there should be no barriers to access for medically necessary services. In effect, the Canada Health Act provided a framework within which 13 disparate provincial and territorial single-payer Medicare systems could continue to evolve yet still provide Canadians with common coverage entitlements (Canada 2002; Maioni 2004).

During the past 15 years, stop-go financing of public health care in Canada has deeply influenced the recent reform process. The first phase was marked by public fiscal constraint in an era of high government debt, first at the provincial level and then later at the federal level. The second phase was marked by increasing health expenditures influenced by a more buoyant economy and lower public debt (Tuohy 2002; Marchildon 2004b).

By 1987, Canada had the second highest level of per capita health care expenditures in the world as measured in US purchase power parity dollars (Mhatre and Deber 1992). The federal and provincial governments combined had accumulated one of the highest public debt loads in the OECD. By the time of the recession of the early 1990s, provincial governments were putting the brakes on health care spending. At the same time, the federal government had frozen its social policy (including health) transfers to the provinces and then, in 1995, announced that it would actually cut transfers to the provinces.

Beginning in 1997, public fiscal restraint was abandoned in favour of increased public spending and tax cuts. Health care expenditures rebounded after years of austerity. As spending grew, however, concerns about the fiscal sustainability of public health care rose, and a lively debate arose concerning the alleged need for new sources of private finance to supplement public finance.

The stop-go aspect is evident from the inflation-adjusted health expenditure data in Table 3.4. From 1991 to 1995, the average real annual growth rate in hospital and physician services (a proxy for insured services under the Canada Health Act) was -0.5%, a consequence of the provinces putting the brakes on health spending to an extent largely unmatched among OECD countries. Although real hospital and physician expenditure growth would move up to 2.1% on average in 1996–2000, the real growth rate in all health expenditures would increase from the 1.6% average in 1991–1995, to 4% in the next five years, a consequence of major increases in other health expenditures, particularly prescription drug spending by governments and private health insurers (Morgan 2005).

7.2   Phase one of health reforms, 1988–1996

During the first phase of reforms, most provinces, in the words of one deputy minister of health, were racing two horses simultaneously: a "black horse" of cost-cutting through health facility and human resource rationalization; and a "white horse" of health reform to improve both quality and access through a more thorough integration of services across the health continuum as well as a rebalancing from illness care to "wellness" (Adams 2001).

Cost-cutting was accomplished, in part, through reducing the number of hospital beds (perhaps long overdue in many parts of the country) and health providers. Hospitals were closed, converted or consolidated into larger units as new surgical techniques, and new prescription drug therapies combined with home care, reduced the demand for hospital beds. Since nurses were salaried employees within hospitals, they were directly affected by these changes. In the early 1990s, newly trained and educated nurses found they had no jobs to go to, and many left the profession for other occupations.

Provincial governments along with provider organizations and educational institutions strove to decrease the supply of nurses through various means that included restricting access to education and increasing the time required for education and training. By the time that the need for nurses was beginning to surge again in the late 1990s, the domestic supply of human resources in the health field was straining to meet demand. Between 1993 and 2002, the number of registered nurses declined by 2%, while the number of licensed practical nurses fell by an astounding 27%.

In contrast, the pressure on physicians came mainly through provincial constraints on their income through the fee schedule. While physicians experienced zero growth during these years, one of the principal reasons (beyond the indirect impact of stagnant income) was the one-year increase in general practitioner training (Chan 2002b).

As can be seen in Table 7.1, rationalization of service delivery was accompanied by a structural reorganization through regionalization. At its most basic, regionalization combines a devolution of funding from the provincial government to regional health authorities (RHAs), now made responsible for the allocation of resources based on the health needs of the regional population, with a centralization of delivery management from individual health facilities to the geographically-based RHA (Marriott and Mable 1998).

The creation of RHAs facilitated the horizontal integration of hospitals, which in turn facilitated careful planning in the downsizing of acute care facilities. Such horizontal integration of acute care facilities conferred some potential economies of scale to the more populous RHAs. The main purpose of the regionalization reforms, however, was to gain the benefits of vertical integration, that is, managerially consolidating facilities and providers across the continuum of care into a single administrative organization capable of improving the coordination and continuity of health services including prevention, public health and health promotion activities. As can be seen in Table 7.2, these health reform objectives formed a consistent part of the recommendations in the arm's-length commissions and task forces that delivered their reports to the governments of Quebec, Nova Scotia, Alberta, Ontario, Saskatchewan and British Columbia between 1988 and 1991 (Mhatre and Deber 1992).

Table 7.1   Phase one of health reforms, 1988–1996

Year	Government	Health reforms/ policy changes	Impact
1988	Quebec	Quebec is the first province to begin establishing regional health authorities (RHAs).	Provides first example in country of how geographic-based RHAs will operate in terms of improving allocation of local health resources and better integrating and rationing health services.
1989	Canada	Federal transfer escalator reduced from GNP −2% to GNP −3%.	Further reduces relative federal contribution to provincial health expenditures.
1990	Canada	Federal transfers frozen. This freeze would be extended to 1995.	Freeze has disproportionate impact on wealthier provinces and Ontario becomes a leading advocate of change in transfer system.
1992	Saskatchewan and New Brunswick	Introduction of major regionalization and wellness reforms accompanied by transformation or closure of rural hospitals.	Integrates various health care organizations along with illness prevention and public health services under RHAs, although size of RHAs increased in 2002. Cost-cutting through rationalization of acute facilities including hospital closure.
1993	Alberta, Newfoundland and Prince Edward Island	Introduction of regionalization and wellness reforms.	As in other provinces, RHAs vertically integrated health care organizations while attempting to introduce illness prevention and public health services. Rationalization of acute care services.
1994	All	Canadian Institute for Health Information (CIHI) created in response to National Task Force on Health Information report (1991), approved by F/P/T ministers of health.	In partnership with Statistics Canada, CIHI is responsible for major health databases concerning health spending, health services and human resources, as well as public reports on indicators and population health.
1995	Canada	Unilateral decision by federal government to reduce cash transfers to province and territories through a new Canada Health and Social Transfer mechanism that has no escalator.	Major reduction in federal cash transfers to provinces. By 2000, the clash over "health funding" becomes the dominant federal-provincial issue and continues through the Romanow Commission.
1996	Nova Scotia, British Columbia and Manitoba	Last provinces to implement a regionalized system of health service delivery other than Ontario.	Adopt similar rationale as other provinces to integrating service delivery across diverse health organizations within a single, geographic region.

In 1988, Quebec was the first province to initiate regionalization but by the mid-1990s, virtually every other province in the country had adopted, or was in the process of adopting similar structural reforms. The degree of integration accompanied by the reforms has varied considerably from province to province.

Table 7.2   Arm's-length provincial reports underpinning phase one reforms

Year	Common Name (Jurisdiction)	Report Title	Main Recommendations
1988	The Rochon Commission (Quebec)	*Rapport de la Commission d'enquête sur les services de santé et les services sociaux*	Supports regionalization reforms and decentralization already being implemented. Emphasis on evidence-based decision-making, needs-based funding, improved professional collaboration and primary care reform.
1989	The Gallant Commission (Nova Scotia)	*The report of the Nova Scotia Royal Commission on Health Care – Towards a new strategy*	Shifts priorities to primary care through limiting funding for institutional and physician care. Urges regionalization to improve service integration and resource allocation in future. Recommends a provincial health council.
1989	The Rainbow Commission (Alberta)	*Rainbow report – Our vision for health*	Urges regionalization to shift resources from institutional care to primary care and illness prevention. Recommends some private financing to increase choice and competition and redefinition of insured services.
1990	Ontario Task Force on Health (Ontario)	*Final report of the Task Force on the Use and Provision of Medical Services*	Hospital restructuring to gain cost efficiencies, better health human resource planning, improved health information and health technology assessment and some organizational change.
1990	The Murray report (Saskatchewan)	*Future directions for health care in Saskatchewan*	Regionalization as a means to obtain cost savings, improve service integration, and shift resources for institutional care to primary care and illness prevention services. Changes fee-for-service remuneration for physicians.
1991	The Seaton Commission (British Columbia)	*Closer to home – Report of the British Columbia Royal Commission on Health Care and Costs*	Places resource limits on institutional and physician care and shifts some resources to illness prevention and public health. Recommends regionalization and health council to establish goals and report to public.

However, in the implementation of regionalization, no province has devolved funding for physician remunerations and prescription drugs to RHAs. According to some, this severely limits the ability of RHAs to meet the health needs of their respective populations in an integrated fashion (Lomas 1997; Lewis and Kouri 2004).

To support health services integration, both orders of government strove to improve their health information and data management infrastructures. Towards the end of the first phase, most provinces were investing heavily in health information networks, including initial efforts at establishing electronic health records. In 1994, the federal government in concert with the provinces established the Canadian Institute for Health Information to better understand and diagnose their respective public health systems. CIHI was initially a consolidation of activities from Statistics Canada, health information programmes from Health Canada, the Hospital Medical Records Institute and the MIS (Management Information Systems) group.[11] In partnership with Statistics Canada, CIHI has grown into one of the world's premier health information agencies with extensive databases on health spending, services and human resources.

The first phase of reform came to an end with the introduction of the Canada Health and Social Transfer and, with it, substantial reductions in cash transfers to the provinces, in 1995/1996. The CHST changed the assumptions on which the original federal-provincial Medicare bargain had been struck and precipitated a major struggle between the federal government and the provinces (Yalnizyan 2004a). With no automatic escalator in the new transfer and no cash floor, the country was instead subjected to a series of episodic and unpredictable negotiations producing one-off agreements on escalation that were little more than temporary ceasefires in the continuing war between Ottawa and the provinces (Marchildon 2004b).

The change initiated by the CHST all but derailed the National Forum on Health, a health reform advisory body that the federal government had originally established in October 1994 (see Table 1.4). Already squabbling over the coming transfer cuts, the provinces refused to participate after the federal government refused to allow a premier to co-chair the forum along with the Prime Minister and the federal Minister of Health. The forum was already on a clear track to recommending a more expansive federal role in Pharmacare and home care when the federal government forced the advisory body to wrap up its work earlier than scheduled (Canada 1997).

Despite this, the National Forum on Health did influence Canadian health policy in terms of increasing awareness of the importance of addressing health determinants beyond health care. In the short term, the federal government was influenced by the forum's recommendation to reorganize and refocus its health research agenda, including creating an Aboriginal health institute that would grapple with the dismal health outcomes of Canada's many First Nations, Inuit and Metis communities. In this respect, the forum added profile to an issue that

---

[11] A non-profit corporation dedicated to developing information system guidelines to assist health care decision-makers, the MIS group was originally an amalgamation of the Management Information Systems Project and the National Hospital Productivity Improvement Program (NHPIP). The MIS group was amalgamated into CIHI in 1994.

was already being pursued by Aboriginal organizations throughout the country. In response to the forum's call for a national health information system, the federal government created a federal/provincial/territorial advisory council and eventually Canada Health Infoway in an effort to speed up the development of health information systems throughout the country.

The National Forum on Health also presaged the second phase of reform in Canada by focusing on the national dimensions of the original Medicare bargain. In particular, the forum's call for a cash floor for federal cash transfers as well as its analysis of the gaps in prescription drug coverage and home care would influence subsequent national studies and commissions.

7.3   Phase two of Canadian health reforms, 1997 to present

As summarized in Table 7.3, Canadians are in the midst of the second phase of health reform and, as a consequence, it is too early to describe with any precision the directions it will take. This period is marked by a significant lift in public health expenditures and growing concerns about the fiscal sustainability of public health care. More importantly, some have questioned the assumptions and values underpinning the Canadian model of Medicare and have urged market-based reforms predicated either on private finance or private delivery, to address what they see as the deficiencies of public health care. Although a minority, this group constitutes an influential sector within Canadian society.

With the growth in expenditures as well as the demand for health services, particularly in the acute sector, many provinces suffered from health human resource shortages in certain sectors and for particular professional services. By 2000, waiting lists for elective surgery had grown longer as the demand for certain services such as orthopaedic surgery grew faster than expected. A dramatic increase in the medical use of advanced diagnostic imaging such as CT scans and magnetic resonance imaging (MRI) created a demand that outstripped the available supply of equipment and the medical radiation technologists, sonographers as well as diagnostic radiation and nuclear medicine physicians who operate, maintain and use such technology (CIHI 2003b). This in turn has had a negative impact on the speed of treatment.

Voter and patient dissatisfaction led to action by both orders of government. The federal government had begun to respond by increasing the size of its health transfers to the provinces and territories. At the same time, it began to demand greater accountability from provincial/territorial governments for the funds transferred as well as more visible recognition for its support. This was

Table 7.3   Most recent phase of health reforms

Year	Government	Health reforms/ policy changes	Impact
2000	Canada	Canadian Institutes of Health Research (CIHR)	Medical Research Council replaced by CIHR. New research strategy and increased funding to make Canada one of top five health research nations.
2000	All	September 2000 First Ministers' Accord on Health Care Renewal	Federal cash transfer funding increased. New conditional funding for primary care reform and medical equipment has mixed results. Creation of separate national corporation (Health Infoway) to accelerate integration of new information technology systems, including electronic health records, also has mixed results.
2002	Saskatchewan	The establishment of a provincial Quality Council to facilitate systematic quality improvements in health care administration and delivery	By 2004, beginning to measure and report on quality performance through standardized indicators for Saskatchewan. Use of quality improvement teams to improve quality performance in key areas including primary care, cancer, surgery and chronic disease.
2003	All	First Ministers' Accord on Health Care Renewal focuses on Health Reform Fund for primary care, home care, catastrophic drug coverage and creation of a national Health Council in response to the recommendations of the Romanow Commission	Limited progress on home care and primary health care reform. New investment in advanced diagnostic services. Delays in establishing Health Council but ultimately proceeds without participation of Quebec and Alberta.
2004	Canada	Public Health Agency of Canada established in response to SARS crisis and desire for more effective federal role in public health coordination	Too early to evaluate.
2004	All	First Ministers' Ten-Year Plan to Strengthen Health Care increases federal funding, sets targets for 24/7 primary care coverage and reform, and reduction of waiting times	Too early to evaluate
2005	Prince Edward Island	Elimination of regional health authorities	Too early to evaluate
2005	Ontario	Introduction of local health integration networks to improve continuity and coordination of care across health sectors	Too early to evaluate

consolidated by the first ministers' health accord in September 2000 that tied some funding to specific objectives such as primary health care reform and improving the stock of medical equipment.

By the second phase of reform, provincial governments were responding to patient and voter dissatisfaction by investing heavily in their systems to address human resource and medical equipment shortfalls. At the same time, some governments became concerned about the pace and impact of their earlier reforms. In the spring and summer of 2000, three provinces – Quebec, Saskatchewan and Alberta – established major arm's-length commissions or task forces to provide recommendations to the three provincial governments on the future direction of their reforms (see Table 7.4).

Quebec's Clair Commission was the first to report, suggesting that more private finance was needed in light of demographic ageing – particularly for long-term care and home care. While the Clair Commission agreed with the basic thrust of regionalization, it made a number of recommendations to fine-tune or change aspects of the province's RHA system (Quebec 2000). The report also insisted that the federal government should increase its financial support to the province through a tax point transfer rather than through an increase in the cash transfer.

The next to report was Saskatchewan's Fyke Commission. It recommended that the provincial government increase the pace and depth of the regionalization reforms as well as establish a Health Quality Council to assist the RHAs to improve the quality of care in priority areas. It also urged that no new money should be pumped into the system until further efficiencies were obtained through the rationalization of existing facilities and the implementation of more effective approaches to primary care and illness/injury prevention (Saskatchewan 2001).

The Mazankowski Task Force also supported the direction of Alberta's regionalization reforms, suggesting that the next logical step was to place the budgets for physicians and prescription drugs in the hands of the RHAs. However, the task force did diverge significantly from the Fyke Commission. In its view, there were few if any efficiencies yet to be gained through further vertical integration and horizontal consolidation but argued that encouraging competition among health organizations could deliver greater efficiencies. The task force rejected the notion of public rationing and instead suggested that additional funding for health care should come from individuals in the form of higher premiums and utilization fees. Cost-containment would be best achieved through an expert panel mandated to review and de-list health services (Alberta 2001).

Although the federal government did not order its own commission of inquiry into health care until 2001, one of the standing committees of Canada's appointed Senate began examining the federal role in health care as early as 1999. This committee of the Senate, chaired by Senator Michael Kirby, would produce a series of reports reviewing the state of Canadian health care in a number of areas as well as setting out various policy options for Canadian governments. Delivered in October 2002, the Senate's final report concluded that more money was required for the system. The Senate committee emphasized what it perceived as the gravity of the waiting-list problem, and recommended that governments be subject to care guarantees on waiting times. After highlighting the extent to which federal cash transfer had fallen over two decades, the Senate argued that Ottawa had an obligation to deliver the lion's share of new funding to the provinces by way of a major increase in cash transfers (Senate 2002a).

The funding recommendation was similar to that ultimately made by the Commission on the Future of Health Care in Canada, commonly known as the Romanow Commission (Canada 2002). Established in April 2001, the Romanow Commission was an independent royal commission established by the Prime Minister partly in response to the possibility of provincial reports and studies then being contemplated or prepared that might challenge the federal role in public health care.

After conducting extensive consultations as well as twelve intensive citizen dialogue sessions, the Romanow Commission concluded that the vast majority of Canadians still supported the principle of universal coverage with access based solely on medical need – the fundamental value underpinning the country's traditional Medicare model. At the same time, it became clear that Canadians wanted their governments to pursue greater efficiencies and to exhibit a higher degree of accountability to the public as the ultimate funders and users of Medicare. And contrary to most government, policy expert and provider expectations (Maxwell et al. 2002; Maxwell, Rosell and Forest 2003), the citizen dialogues demonstrated that Canadians were willing to:

- be rostered within a primary care network;
- have their personal health information stored on an electronic health record and shared with health professionals to facilitate and improve service;
- exercise greater responsibility, individually and collectively, to prevent illness and injury as well as to pursue greater health literacy.

The final report of the Romanow Commission recommended a series of changes beyond increased federal funding, including:

- creating a national health council to provide advice to governments and provide progress and performance reports on key aspects of the pan-Canadian reform agenda to the general public;

Table 7.4   **Arm's-length provincial and national reports underpinning phase two reforms, 1997–2004**

Year	Common Name (Jurisdiction)	Report Title	Main Recommendations
1997	National Forum on Health (Canada)	*Canada health action: building on the legacy*	National Pharmacare programme and national home care programme. Recommends increase in investment in health and health care research as well as health information management systems.
2000	The Ontario Health Services Restructuring Commission (Ontario)	*Looking back, looking forward: the Legacy report*	Decision-making mandate to rationalize and close hospitals and advisory role for other health services. Improved health and management information as well as outcomes and performance measurement. More resources for home care and long-term care. Some decentralization urged.
2000	The Clair Commission (Quebec)	*Rapport de la Commission d'étude sur les services de santé et les services sociaux: les solutions emergent*	Limit scope of coverage and seek private capital finance options including P3s. More federal financial support through tax point transfer. Improve recruitment and retention of health human resources. Renew commitment to regionalization but with some organizational change.
2001	The Fyke Commission (Saskatchewan)	*Caring for Medicare: sustaining a quality system*	Establish Quality Council to improve outcomes. Reduce number of small (rural) hospitals for reasons of cost and quality. Accelerate primary health care through provider teams and alternative physician remuneration.
2002	The Mazankowski Task Force (Alberta)	*A framework for reform: report of the Premier's Advisory Council on Health*	More private users pay in place of further public rationing. More choice of provider and competition among health organizations. Increase devolution from provincial government to regions. Expert panel for de-listing services. Accelerate primary care reform.
2002	The Kirby Committee (Canada)	*The health of Canadians – the federal role: recommendations for reform by the Standing Senate Committee on Social Affairs, Science and Technology*	Increase federal funding. Improve primary care, expand home care and introduce catastrophic drug coverage. Change hospital funding to needs/service-based funding. Care guarantees to shock governments into addressing waiting lists. More health research.
2002	The Romanow Commission (Canada)	*Building on values: the future of health care in Canada*	Redefining federal role. Increased federal transfer funding to provinces. Accelerate primary care changes. Expand home care to include mental health as well as post-acute and palliative care. Establish National Drug Agency, national drug formulary, catastrophic drug coverage and medication management. Consolidate funding and experiment with Aboriginal Health Partnerships.
2003	National Advisory Committee on SARS and Public Health (Canada)	*Learning from SARS: renewal of public health in Canada*	Increase federal investment in public health infrastructure. Creation of national public health agency. Improve disease surveillance systems and epidemic response capacity.

- updating, clarifying and strengthening the Canada Health Act;
- creating a national platform for targeted home care services for mental health, post-acute care, and palliative care;
- pushing primary health care and prevention to the centre stage of the Canadian health system including a national immunization strategy;
- providing catastrophic prescription drug coverage and addressing current prescription and utilization patterns through improved medication management;
- creating a National Drug Agency to regulate the prices of prescription and generic drugs, and establishing a national drug formulary;
- focusing on the access and quality of care challenges faced by rural and remote communities through training, education and the improvement of infrastructure;
- addressing the fragmentation of Aboriginal health care funding and delivery and its cultural relevance through integrated Aboriginal health organizations.

So far, at least some of the recommendations from the most recent crop of provincial reports have been implemented. In Ontario, the provincial government has moved in the direction of decentralizing the allocation of resources while integrating health delivery through local health integration networks. In Saskatchewan, a health quality council was established. In Alberta, despite some threats to the contrary, the provincial government has not introduced utilization fees or medical savings accounts, both of which would violate the accessibility principle, and trigger the penalties for extra charges and user fees under the Canada Health Act.

In response to the national and provincial reports, federal, provincial and territorial governments negotiated a consensus concerning the priority areas for national health reform. In the 2003 First Ministers' Accord on Health Care Renewal, the country's premiers and Prime Minister focused on accelerating primary care and home care reform as well as the development of electronic health records. They also sought to improve catastrophic drug coverage and advanced diagnostic services (CICS 2003). To review progress, all governments, with the exceptions of Quebec and Alberta, agreed to establish the Health Council of Canada. The Romanow report had recommended a segregated, cash-only federal transfer for health care to encourage greater transparency in future federal-provincial negotiations over health care funding. While the federal government split the Canada Health and Social Transfer into two separate transfers – a Canada Social Transfer and a Canada Health Transfer – it did not eliminate the tax transfer portion (McIntosh 2004).

In response to the National Advisory Committee on SARS and Public Health, the federal government established the Public Health Agency of Canada. At the same time, the federal government increased its direct expenditures on public health infrastructure, including bolstering its disease surveillance and epidemic response capacities.

In the 2004 Ten-Year Plan to Strengthen Health Care, first ministers agreed to develop benchmarks and comparable indicators for public reporting on waiting times, and targeted reductions in waiting times in five priority areas (cancer, cardiac, diagnostic imaging, sight restoration and joint replacement). The federal government also agreed to provide C$5.5 billion over 10 years through a Wait Time Reduction Fund to assist provinces and territories to increase access by reducing wait times.

First ministers also agreed to target home care changes in three areas: post-acute, mental health and end-of-life. In terms of primary care, all governments said they would commit to providing at least 50% of their populations with 24/7 access to multidisciplinary teams by 2011. The federal government also increased its funding to territorial governments and Aboriginal organizations in order to facilitate reform and improve access, including medical transportation infrastructure for remote northern communities. With the exception of Quebec, both orders of government created a ministerial task force to work on a national pharmaceutical strategy (CICS 2004; Marchildon 2005).

In taking these actions, governments have begun to implement many of the recommendations contained in national and provincial reports since 1997. At the same time, however, some issues remain largely unaddressed, including the regulation and growing cost of prescription drugs as well as the impact of the highly fragmented system of Aboriginal health care.

8. Assessment of the health system

8.1 Assessing the components: public, mixed and private

The Canadian health system is best described as an amalgam of public, mixed and private systems of health care. The universal part of the public health care system is made up of 13 separate single-payer universal schemes held together by some broad standards set out in the Canada Health Act and enforced by federal transfers and potential penalties. Public coverage is deep (no user fees) but also very narrow, as the core of Medicare remains hospital and physician services though most primary care and public health services are also included by the provinces.

Hospital and physician services alone constitute almost 43% of total health expenditures, but if direct federal expenditures for public health, health research, health and prescription drug regulation, illness prevention and health promotion initiatives along with coverage and services for First Nations people, Inuit, the Royal Canadian Mounted Police, the armed forces and veterans are included in a slightly broader definition of Medicare, then the total of these services would be close to 50% of total health expenditures in Canada (CIHI 2004d).

Although Medicare varies somewhat in terms of access, coverage and quality across the country, the provincial/territorial differences are held in check through the national framework provided by the Canada Health Act. As a consequence, it is possible to make some assessments of this public "system" on an aggregated national basis.

Table 8.1   Public, mixed and private systems of health care

	Funding	Administration	Delivery
Public Canada Health Act services (hospital and physician services plus) and public health services	Public taxation	Universal, single-payer provincial systems. Private self-regulating professions subject to provincial legislative framework	Private professional, private not-for-profit, private-for-profit and public arm's-length facilities and organizations
Mixed goods and services, including most prescription drugs, home care and institutional care services	Public taxation, private insurance and out-of-pocket payments	Public services that are generally welfare-based and targeted, private services regulated in the public interest by governments	Private professional, private not-for-profit and for-profit, and public arm's length facilities and organizations
Private goods and services including most dental and vision care as well as over-the-counter drugs and alternative medicines	Private insurance and out-of-pocket payments including full payments, co-payments and deductibles	Private ownership and control; private professions, some self-regulating with public regulation of food, drugs and natural health products.	Private providers and private-for-profit facilities and organizations

Source: Adapted from Marchildon 2004c.

As the name suggests, the mixed system refers to the public and private funding, administration and delivery that apply to home care, non-hospital institutional care and most prescription drugs. To the extent that there is public coverage or subsidy for these health services and goods, it varies considerably across the ten provinces and three territories. Moreover, the private means of funding, administration and delivery of these services have also evolved differently in the different provinces and territories. Both these factors make any national assessments of the mixed "system" difficult if not misleading. It is none the less useful to compare the aggregate outcomes produced by this important part of the Canadian system to other countries, particularly those countries in which many health services are relatively decentralized such as Australia, Sweden and the United States.

Beyond these mixed services and goods, there is a large sector of health goods and services that are almost entirely provided through private funding and delivery. These include most dental and vision care as well as alternative medical therapies and over-the-counter medication. Together, these mixed and private systems of health constitute approximately 50% of total health expenditures.

8.2   Assessing the public (Medicare) health sector

According to the Canada Health Act (1984), the principal objective of the provincial and territorial Medicare systems is to deliver medically necessary or medically required services on a universal basis without financial obstacles of any kind. Judged by these objectives, the Canadian system has performed quite well. The basket of services covered under this definition has grown with improvements in medical technologies and knowledge. More surprising perhaps, provinces and territories have produced remarkably similar coverage for their residents despite the lack of specificity concerning any common basket of Medicare services in the federal legislation. With some exceptions, universality in the sense of all Canadians obtaining Medicare on the same terms and conditions has been upheld. Finally, and again with few exceptions, access to medically necessary or required services has been on the basis of need rather than ability to pay.

In recent years, the focus of Canadians has shifted from financial barriers to access (which had largely disappeared by virtue of the elimination of most user fees under Medicare) to non-financial barriers to access, in particular the question of timely access to health care. These barriers to access have included waiting lists for certain diagnostic tests and surgical procedures as well as access to certain types of specialist physicians, or even family physicians, in some parts of the country.

The Mazankowski report for the provincial Government of Alberta questioned the manner in which the provincial and territorial health organizations have rationed health services, and the final report of the Senate Committee recommended the imposition of minimum waiting times through financially binding care guarantees on the provinces and territories (Alberta 2001, Senate 2002). No government has yet imposed upon itself or others such binding care guarantees.

The other approach is for individuals or interest groups to use the courts to impose a standard of care quality or timeliness on government. Greschner (2004) and Jackman (2004) provide a survey of constitutional cases launched by litigants in an effort to reshape the way governments administer and deliver Medicare. Until recently, most of these cases were unsuccessful, leaving governments largely free to determine how public health care services should be funded, administered and delivered as well as the dividing line between public (Medicare) and private sector in health services.

In 2005, however, in the case of *Chaoulli* v. *Quebec*, the Supreme Court of Canada decided that the Government of Quebec's prohibition on private health insurance was contrary to that province's Charter of Human Rights and Freedoms in a situation when an individual's lengthy wait for Medicare services seriously compromises the health of that individual. The Supreme Court gave the Government of Quebec a year to make its Medicare law consistent with its own charter.

Although a bare majority of Supreme Court justices concluded that the facts in the *Chaoulli* case did not involve an infringement of right to life, liberty, or security of the person under the Canadian Charter of Rights and Freedoms, the other five provinces (British Columbia, Alberta, Manitoba, Ontario and Prince Edward Island) with express prohibitions on private Medicare insurance are reviewing their own laws in anticipation of possible constitutional litigation in the near future. From a broader political standpoint, the *Chaoulli* v. *Quebec* decision has raised a fundamental challenge to the Canadian model of single-payer Medicare.

At the same time, the single-payer health insurance system has some undeniable advantages. In terms of the cost of public health care, Canada is among the higher-cost OECD countries. At the same time, however, the country's public health care costs per capita are lower than public health care costs in the United States even without taking into consideration tax expenditure subsidies that are a major factor in the US system. This is a result of the lower administrative costs associated with a single-payer public insurance system relative to the high administrative costs associated with a private multi-payer system (Mossialos and Dixon 2002; Evans 2004). Having a single payer such as a provincial government administer the system means that substantial resources are saved in terms of the billing, contracting, bill collecting and marketing, as well as the infrastructure required to assess risk, set premiums and design complex benefit packages associated with a competitive private insurance environment. In a recent estimate based upon 1999 data, Canadian administrative costs were calculated at $325 per capita, while those in the United States were estimated to be C$1151, well over three times the costs in Canada (Woolhandler et al. 2003).

While the evidence of administrative efficiency seems compelling, a few commentators and experts have questioned the single-payer administrative model, albeit less on the basis of efficiency grounds than on the basis of freedom of choice in terms of differing insurance benefits (Gratzer 1999, 2002; Hussey and Anderson 2003). With one possible exception, there is little debate concerning the merits of continuing with a single-payer model for Medicare services. Despite the extra cost involved in private insurance, the Mazankowski report recommended that the Government of Alberta consider breaking down the "monopoly" of the single-payer system, and possibly allowing some competition through private insurance (Alberta 2001). Thus far, however, the Government of Alberta has not moved to refashion its single-payer model into a multi-payer insurance system.

Primary health care has been at the centre of the Medicare reform agenda since the 1960s (Hastings 1972). As the most common first point of contact with the health system, primary care has also been viewed as the lynch pin between Canada Health Act services and health care services not covered by the legislation, from prescription drug therapy to home and long-term care. For provincial governments, improving primary care has also been an important element in their recent efforts to encourage a shift of some resources from higher-cost acute and institutional care to lower-cost home and community care (Wilson, Shortt and Dorland 2004).

According to Hutchison, Abelson and Lavis (2001), there have been three waves of primary care reform at the provincial level. In the 1970s, provinces developed alternative models of organization and funding; in the 1980s, they began to expand the scope of providers; and by the mid-1990s, they were beginning to launch numerous pilot projects. Since about 2000, however, the pace of primary care reform has picked up considerably in Canada, aided in part by new funding earmarked for primary care in the first ministers' agreements of 2000, 2003, and 2004. In addition, the Primary Health Care Transition Fund administered by Health Canada supported the development of tools and indicators to evaluate primary health care initiatives (Tuohy 2004; CICS 2000, 2003). As of 2004, however, no comprehensive national assessment of primary care reform had been conducted in Canada (Wilson, Shortt and Dorland 2004).

Regionalization may eventually change the dynamics of primary care reform in Canada. At this point, no regional health authority (RHA) has control over physician remuneration or prescription drug funding and administration. Two recent provincial commissions advised that RHAs be given control over the former (and hinted at the latter) in order to give them greater flexibility in developing primary health care initiatives, including the replacement of fee-schedule remuneration with alternative payment schemes for physicians (Saskatchewan 2001; Alberta 2001).

Regionalization has changed Medicare by more effectively integrating hospital, physician and associated services covered under the Canada Health Act (CHA) with those provincially covered or subsidized health services that are not part of the CHA. However, although a comprehensive and systematic study of the impact of regionalization has not been carried out, some concerns have been raised about the benefits of regionalization, particularly in terms of whether it has produced a positive shift in resources from downstream curative activities to upstream illness prevention and health promotion activities (McFarlane and Prado 2002).

In 2005, the least populous province in Canada – Prince Edward Island – abandoned its regionalized structure of health services. At the same time, Canada's most populous province, Ontario, has adopted a form of regionalization through the establishment of local health integration networks under a mandate that resembles the one given to regional health authorities in a number of other provinces. Indeed, two long-time health system experts have argued that the future of a regionalized system of health organization and delivery seems relatively secure in most provinces (Lewis and Kouri 2004).

The stop-go financing of health care by governments during the last 15 years has created disruptions on a number of fronts including some damage to public confidence in the ability of governments to manage public health care, particularly at the intergovernmental level; recurring concern about the future sustainability of the system, and, at least by the end of the 1990s, rising concerns about the length of waiting times for some services. A political challenge for provincial and territorial governments and a managerial challenge for regional health authorities, hospitals and medical practitioners, waiting lists are now commonly perceived as the "Achilles' heel of Canadian Medicare" (Noseworthy et al. 2003).

The Western Canada Waiting List Project was established in 1999 to develop priority-setting scoring tools for waiting lists in five clinical areas: cataract surgery; general surgery procedures; hip and knee replacement; magnetic resonance imaging (MRI); and children's mental health (Hadorn et al. 2000). Based in part on the approach pioneered by the Western Canada Waiting List Project, the Saskatchewan Surgical Care Network was established in 2002 to plan and manage surgical services in the province as well as develop standards, monitor performance and communicate with patients and health providers on surgical access. In addition, best practices in waiting list management were identified as a priority to be addressed by federal, provincial and territorial governments in the First Ministers' Health Summit of 2004 (CICS 2004).

In 2005, the Western Canada Waiting List Project released a set of "maximum acceptable waiting times" that it had developed using public, patient and clinical input, and then linked to levels of urgency based upon priority criteria scores. This work partially influenced the Canadian Medical Association's report on waiting time benchmarks (CMA 2005).

8.3   Beyond Medicare: assessing the mixed health sector

In contrast to Medicare, very little attention has been devoted to assessing the performance of the mixed health sector in Canada as a whole. In addition, only limited attention has been paid to assessing the individual sectors within the mixed system from community care, including long-term care and home care, to the relative performance of provincial prescription drug plans.

In terms of the various programmes and policies that make up the spectrum of services embraced by the phrase "community care", there has been little effort to standardize definitional categories so that provincial services can be usefully contrasted and compared much less assessed in terms of performance, although the Canadian Institute for Health Information and Statistics Canada have begun the job of establishing the definitional criteria for proper data collection and analysis.

Since 2001, the Canadian Institute for Health Information has published an annual compendium on national, provincial and territorial drug expenditure trends (CIHI 2003d). Although it is difficult to make systematic comparisons because of definitional differences, it is clear that Canada is much closer to the United States than it is to the other comparator countries in terms of its reliance on private funding for drugs. Public drug expenditures as a percentage of total drug expenditures in Canada are 36.1% compared to 53.7% in Australia and 65.9% in France (CIHI 2003d). Since private sector drug plans are generally unavailable to the working poor, many of whom may also be excluded from public drug coverage, this probably reflects a serious problem of access.

Despite their growing importance, long-term care and home care have received relatively limited scholarly attention, at least from a health system's perspective as opposed to a clinical perspective. Future improvements in the coordination and continuity of care will depend heavily on evidence-based analyses that systematically examine long-term and home care programmes and policies across Canada but such an initiative would probably have to be taken at an intergovernmental level to produce meaningful comparisons.

8.4   Assessing the private health sector

In part because of the absence of public funding, there has been no systematic study of the efficient or effective performance of the private health sector on an aggregate basis. Similarly, while there have been few independent studies of individual private health service sectors (for instance, Baldota and Leake 2004, for dentistry), there have been no major national studies of these sectors, or the private health sector as a whole, in recent years.

In contrast, there has been some study of private-for-profit delivery within the publicly-administered part of health care (Deber 2004). In particular, a debate has raged concerning the impact of replacing public or private not-for-profit health care organizations with private-for-profit firms on efficiency, effectiveness, choice and access in terms of the current public system (Devereaux et al. 2004; Gratzer 2002; Ramsay 2004).

A number of private services are actually supported or subsidized through public finance but the nature and size of this public commitment is largely unknown. As a consequence, a national initiative examining tax expenditure subsidies for health services would be very useful. In addition, a pan-Canadian study of the impact of provincial workers' compensation systems with single-payer Medicare systems would be of considerable utility.

8.5   Overall health status and health indicator performance

Health status and health system indicators must be carefully selected when comparing performance of national health systems. In particular, health status can be more influenced by broader determinants such as living and working conditions, personal and community resources and environmental factors than by access to, and the performance of, a given health system.

Despite these serious limitations, it is useful to examine the Canadian population's position relative to Australia, France, Sweden, the United Kingdom and the United States. Sweden generally performs in the top rank of OECD countries on many of the basic determinants of health. As Table 8.2 illustrates, this translates into higher than average life expectancy and lower mortality rates for Sweden. It is interesting to note, however, that both Canada and Australia rank consistently high on these indicators, much higher than the United States and the United Kingdom. When it comes to immunization rates – reasonable indicators concerning the effectiveness of public and primary health care – Canada ranks high for measles immunization but low for diphtheria/tetanus/pertussis (DPT) immunization.

While health status rankings reveal the relative health of a population, they do not provide a measure of a health system's actual performance. For this, it is necessary to find measures of either processes or outcomes of care that are linked

Table 8.2   Health status indicator relative rankings, 2000 (overall OECD rankings in brackets)

	Life expectancy at birth	Potential years of life lost per 100 000	Perinatal mortality per 100 000	DPT immunization % of children	Measles immunization % of children
Australia	3 (7)	3 (8)	2 (8)	4 (14)	3 (16)
Canada	2 (5)	2 (7)	3 (11)	5 (19)	1 (7)
France	4 (8)	5 (18)	4 (16)	2 (5)	6 (24)
Sweden	1 (4)	1 (1)	1 (7)	1 (2)	2 (8)
United Kingdom	5 (18)	4 (12)	5 (17)	3 (13)	4 (15)
United States	6 (20)	6 (24)	6 (18)	6 (20)	5 (19)

Source: Derived from OECD 2004a.

Note: 2000 has been used as a base year due to unavailability of data for OECD countries after that year. Figures for 1999 have been used in some cases for France and the United Kingdom. For the first three columns, a lower mortality figure for a given country produces a higher relative ranking.

to public health care policies or delivery features, although population health factors continue to play an important role. Table 8.3 picks out a very few of the potentially large number of indicators based upon this factor. While too small a set of indicators to allow strong conclusions to be drawn, Canada's performance relative to Australia, France, Sweden, the United Kingdom and the United States varies from very good to mediocre. It is excellent for cerebrovascular diseases, good to average for ischaemic heart and respiratory diseases, and average to mediocre in the treatment of cancer (malignant neoplasms).

An indicator of health status that is directly connected to the quality of health care systems is avoidable mortality, or mortality amenable to medical/health care. In the comparative study by Nolte and McKee (2003) using an aggregate

Table 8.3   Disease mortality indicator relative rankings, 2000 (overall OECD rankings in brackets)

	Malignant neoplasms	Cerebrovascular diseases	Respiratory system diseases	Ischaemic heart diseases
Australia	2 (8)	4 (5)	4 (12)	2 (11)
Canada	4 (15)	1 (2)	3 (10)	3 (12)
France	5 (18)	2 (3)	2 (8)	1 (3)
Sweden	1 (2)	5 (11)	1 (4)	4 (16)
United Kingdom	6 (20)	6 (18)	6 (25)	6 (22)
United States	3 (14)	3 (4)	5 (22)	5 (21)

Source: Derived from OECD 2004a.
Note: 2000 has been used as a base year due to the unavailability of data for OECD countries after that year.

measure of avoidable mortality, Canada ranked fourth among 19 OECD countries, behind Sweden and Australia but ahead of France, the United States and the United Kingdom.

Although these results provide a view of where Canada sits relative to other advanced industrial countries in terms of health and health care, these results must be treated with considerable caution. First, they provide a comparison at one static point in time. Second, mere rankings do not indicate the extent of the spread among countries in terms of an individual indicator. Third, differences in data collection and quality among countries may produce skewed results.

More detailed studies of a single indicator are ultimately more useful in determining differences in health quality. In two recent studies of differences in survival rates for various types of cancer, for example, researchers discovered that there were no significant differences between Canadians and Americans except at the lower socioeconomic status end of the spectrum. In particular, low-income cancer patients in Toronto enjoyed a much higher survival rate than their counterparts in Detroit and Honolulu (Gorey et al. 1997, 2000). Although the study is limited to three urban areas, the results at least suggest that Ontario's (and by extension Canada's) more equitable access to preventive and therapeutic health care through its single-payer universal system is responsible for the significant difference in outcomes.

At the same time, there is some evidence that the reinvestment in public health care that began in 1997 is beginning to have a positive impact on the average patient's perception of the timeliness and quality of care. Based upon two Canadian Community Health Surveys conducted by Statistics Canada, individuals who had received hospital, physician, community-based or telehealth services – all predominantly public health care services – in the preceding 12 calendar months, were asked to report on their relative level of satisfaction or dissatisfaction with these services. Table 8.4 illustrates a positive trend upwards overall in the country as well in the majority of provinces and territories.

While all of the "performance" indicators discussed above can shed only limited light on the Canadian health system, they should at least demonstrate that public health care is not in crisis. While there is room for much improvement, Canada is faring reasonably well relative to other OECD countries on at least some key indicators. In addition, the individuals who actually use the system are becoming more, rather than less, satisfied with public health care.

Table 8.4   Patient satisfaction with public health care, 2001 and 2003

	2001 % excellent or good	2003 % excellent or good
British Columbia	84.0	82.8
Alberta	83.6	85.7
Saskatchewan	85.6	88.4
Manitoba	80.3	85.6
Ontario	84.5	87.1
Quebec	85.0	89.0
New Brunswick	82.8	86.9
Nova Scotia	85.3	87.3
Prince Edward Island	89.6	88.6
Newfoundland and Labrador	88.9	86.1
Yukon	81.7	85.3
Northwest Territories	80.5	79.1
Nunavut	70.8	77.1
Canada	**84.4**	**86.8**

Source: Statistics Canada. *Health Indicators.* Vol. 2005, No. 2: June 2005.

Note: The results were based on Canadian Community Health Surveys conducted by Statistics Canada in which those surveyed were asked: "Overall, how would you rate the quality of the health care you received? Would you say it was: excellent, good, fair or poor?".

9. Conclusions

Before the introduction of national hospitalization and national Medicare, Canadian health care was on a trajectory parallel to that of the United States (Maioni 1998). The introduction of provincial and territorial single-payer systems in the provinces for hospital and physician services, and the subsequent passage of the Canada Health Act (1984), has produced a system which is broadly comparable to the universal systems of western Europe. In this sense, Canada has evolved very differently from the United States, although the mixed and private portions of the Canadian system as opposed to the public – Medicare – portion, have strong institutional similarities with the American system (Maioni 1998; Tuohy 1999).

In terms of mortality data that can be related to medical care, it is important to note that Canada ranks well above the United States and the United Kingdom (Nolte and McKee 2003), and other evidence indicates that public health spending has had an appreciable impact on Canadian mortality outcomes (Laporte and Ferguson 2003).

Despite growing public dissatisfaction with aspects of the system in the 1990s, in part spurred by deep public funding cutbacks early in the decade, most Canadians remain committed to the fundamental working principles of Medicare, including public administration and universality, although debate continues concerning the role of private-for-profit firms in the delivery of health care services within Medicare (Deber 2004). Due to the presence of numerous not-for-profit and arm's-length institutions that are not directly managed by government, the Canadian context for this debate is different from countries where governments actually have held a monopoly over the delivery of public health care services. The introduction of "market forces" into provincial single-payer delivery systems can be seen in the contracting-out of ancillary services as well as the planning and construction of public–private-partnership health facilities, including hospitals, in Alberta, British Columbia, Ontario and Quebec.

There has been greater consensus on the need to achieve greater administrative efficiency and service quality. Governments at both levels have improved the quality and breadth of health research and data collection, introduced performance measurement and more systematic health technology assessment, more thorough quality management and patient safety protocols. Recently, governments have devoted increasing resources to improving access by improving waiting-list management and, where possible, devoting new resources to reduce or eliminate bottlenecks in the delivery of services. Their concerns are directly related to patient dissatisfaction with the performance of Medicare on this front and their collective desire to restore the public's confidence in the system. Since these efforts are relatively new, and some are at a very experimental stage, it will take years to determine their relative success.

As the first point of contact to the health care system for most Canadians, primary health services are a critical determinant of access. Aided by recent federal health transfer increases, the provinces and territories are currently engaged in a series of primary care reforms that vary considerably from jurisdiction to jurisdiction, particularly in terms of the role of the physician relative to other health providers. Whether the pace of reforming primary care will slow down in the same way as past efforts remains to be seen.

Some critical areas of health care policy remain unaddressed. On the public health front, much more could be done in terms of public health interventions and education, given the fact that the number of deaths attributed to overweight and obesity soared between 1985 and 2000 (Katzmarzyk and Ardern 2004). The same argument can be applied to the high incidence of diabetes among Aboriginal Canadians.

In terms of access and coverage, provincial and territorial drug plans form an uneven patchwork quilt in Canada. Rising costs are already creating a crisis of sustainability for many of the programmes yet little is being done to address prescription and utilization behaviours in a thorough manner. Despite the fact that the federal government has considerable regulatory jurisdiction, as well as bargaining leverage that far exceeds any individual province in terms of the pharmaceutical industry, there has been little discussion about the possibility of radical policy alternatives to the status quo. One such possibility would be for the provinces to agree to allow the federal government to finance and administer a national drug programme similar to the Pharmaceutical Benefits Scheme in Australia.

There has been much discussion surrounding the importance of home care services in providing more appropriate and higher-quality care that is often less costly than institutional care in hospitals and nursing homes. To achieve meaningful change, the federal government should consider adding post-acute home care, home mental health and palliative care services to the Canada Health Act (Canada 2002). An ageing population combined with a sharp increase in brain disorders such as dementia and delirium will none the less require new public and private investments in long-term care. Despite this, little is known about the administration and delivery of long-term care in Canada. As a consequence, it would be timely and useful to have a national commission examine long-term care to provide a solid foundation for policy change in this critical area.

In the 1980s, Canadians were, by far, more satisfied with their health system than other comparator OECD countries. To regain this level of satisfaction, governments and health organizations must be prepared to initiate major reforms – some of which will threaten existing stakeholders as well as change the scope of practice boundaries for providers – and invest more public money. At the same time, based upon the evidence of major health surveys, most Canadians have been experiencing some improvement in the quality and timeliness of their services in recent years.

10. References

Abelson J, Mendelson M, Lavis JN, Morgan SG, Forest PG. Canadians confront health care reform. *Health Affairs*, 2004, 23(3):186–193.

Adams D. Canadian federalism and the development of national health goals and objectives. In: Adams D, ed. *Federalism, democracy and health policy in Canada*. Montreal and Kingston, McGill-Queen's University Press, 2001:61–105.

Agriculture and Agri-Food Canada. *Canadian rural population trends*. Ottawa, Agriculture and Agri-Food Canada, 2002 (AAFC publication number 2138/E).

Alberta. *Rainbow report – Our vision for health*. Two volumes. Edmonton, Premier's Commission on Future Health Care for Albertans, 1989.

Alberta. *A framework for reform. Report of the Premier's Advisory Council on Health* [D Mazankowsi, Chair]. Edmonton, Premier's Advisory Council on Health, 2001.

Alberta. *A sustainable health system for Alberta. Report of the MLA Task Force on Health Care Funding and Revenue Generation*. Edmonton, Alberta Health and Wellness, 2002.

Anis, AH. Pharmaceutical policies in Canada: Another example of federal-provincial discord. *Canadian Medical Association Journal*, 2000, 162(4):523–526.

Association of Workers' Compensation Boards of Canada. *Shared responsibility: workers' compensation and the future of health care in Canada*. Ottawa. Submission to the Commission on the Future of Health Care in Canada, 2001.

Auerbach L, Donner A, Peters DD, Townson M, Yalnizyan A. *Funding hospital infrastructure: why P3s don't work, and what will*. Ottawa, Canadian Centre for Policy Alternatives, 2003.

Baldota K, Leake J. A macroeconomic review of dentistry in Canada in the 1990s. *Journal of the Canadian Dental Association*, 2004, 70(9):604–609.

Ballinger G, Zhang J, Hicks V. *Home care estimates in national health care expenditures*. Ottawa, Canadian Institute for Health Information, 2001.

Barer ML, Morgan SG, Evans RG. Strangulation or rationalization? Cost and access in Canadian hospitals. *Longwoods Review*, 2004, 1(4):10–19.

Bégin M. *Medicare: Canada's right to health*. Ottawa, Optimum Publishing, 1988.

Bourgeault IL. Delivering the "new" Canadian midwifery. The impact on midwifery of integration into the Ontario health system. *Sociology of Health and Illness*, 2000, 22(2):172–196.

Boychuk T. *The making and meaning of hospital policy in the United States and Canada*. Ann Arbor, University of Michigan Press, 1999.

Braën A. Health and the distribution of powers in Canada. In: McIntosh T, Forest PG, Marchildon GP, eds. *The governance of health care in Canada*. Toronto, University of Toronto Press, 2004:25–49.

British Columbia. *Closer to home: Report of the British Columbia Commission on Health Care and Costs* [P Seaton, Chair]. Victoria, BC, British Columbia Commission on Health Care and Costs, 1991.

British Columbia. *2003/2004 Report 4. Alternative payments to physicians: a program in need of change*. Vancouver, Office of the Auditor-General of British Columbia, 2003.

Canada. *Report of the Royal Commission on Aboriginal Peoples. Volumes 1-5* [R Dussault and G Erasmus, Co-Chairs]. Ottawa, Royal Commission on Aboriginal Peoples, 1996.

Canada. *Royal Commission on Health Services: Volume I*. Ottawa, Queen's Printer, 1964.

Canada. *Canada health action: building the legacy. Vol. I-II. The final report of the National Forum on Health*. Ottawa, National Forum on Health, 1997.

Canada. *Building on values: the future of health care in Canada* [RJ Romanow, Commissioner]. Saskatoon, Commission on the Future of Health Care in Canada, 2002.

Canada Health Infoway. *EHRS blueprint. An interoperable HER framework*. Montreal, Canada Health Infoway Inc., 2003.

Canadian Alliance of Physiotherapy Regulators and the Canadian Physiotherapy Association. *Physiotherapy health human resources. Background paper.* Submission to Health Canada, 2002.

Canadian Association of Occupational Therapists. *Profile of occupational therapy practice in Canada, second edition.* Ottawa, Canadian Association of Occupational Therapists, 2002.

Canadian Centre for the Analysis of Regionalization and Health. Updated provincial tables on regionalization (http://www.regionalization.org, 2004).

Canadian Life and Health Insurance Association. *The role of supplementary health insurance in Canada's health system.* Toronto. Submission to the Commission on the Future of Health Care in Canada, 2001.

Canadian Nurses Advisory Committee. *Our health, our future. Creating quality workplaces for Canadian nurses.* Ottawa, Health Canada for the Federal/ Provincial/Territorial Ministers of Health Advisory Committee on Health Human Resources, 2002.

Casey JT. *Status report and analysis of health professional regulations in Canada.* Prepared for the Federal/Provincial/Territorial Ministers of Health Advisory Committee on Health Human Resources. Edmonton, Field Atkinson Perraton, 1999.

Caulfield T. Medical malpractice, the common law, and health-care reform. In: Marchildon GP, McIntosh T, Forest PG, eds. *The fiscal sustainability of health care in Canada.* Toronto, University of Toronto Press, 2004:81–109.

Chan B. *From perceived surplus to perceived shortage. What happened to Canada's physician workforce in the 1990s?* Ottawa, Canadian Institute for Health Information, 2002a.

Chan B. The declining comprehensiveness of primary care. *Canada Medical Association Journal*, 2002b, 166(4):429–434.

CICS. *2000 First Ministers' Accord on Health Care Renewal.* Ottawa, Canadian Intergovernmental Conference Secretariat, 11 September 2000.

CICS. *2003 First Ministers' Accord on Health Care Renewal.* Ottawa, Canadian Intergovernmental Conference Secretariat, 4 February 2003.

CICS. *A Ten-Year Plan to Strengthen Health Care.* Ottawa, Canadian Intergovernmental Conference Secretariat, 16 September 2004.

CIHI. Discharge abstract database. Ottawa, Canadian Institute for Health Information (http://secure.cihi.ca/cihiweb/dispPage.jsp?cw_page=services_dad_e, accessed 5 August 2005).

CIHI. Hospital morbidity database. Ottawa, Canadian Institute for Health Information (http://secure.cihi.ca/cihiweb/dispPage.jsp?cw_page=service_hmdb_e, accessed 5 August 2005).

CIHI. *Canada's health care providers*. Ottawa, Canadian Institute for Health Information, 2001.

CIHI. *Supply, distribution and migration of Canadian physicians*. Ottawa, Canadian Institute for Health Information, 2002.

CIHI. *National health expenditure trends, 1975–2003*. Ottawa, Canadian Institute for Health Information, 2003a.

CIHI. *Medical imaging in Canada*. Ottawa, Canadian Institute for Health Information, 2003b.

CIHI. *Hospital report 2003: acute care*. Ottawa, Canadian Institute for Health Information, 2003c.

CIHI. *Drug expenditure in Canada, 1975–2003*. Ottawa, Canadian Institute for Health Information, 2003d.

CIHI. *Improving the health of Canadians*. Ottawa, Canadian Institute for Health Information, 2004a.

CIHI. *Health personnel trends in Canada, 1993–2002*. Ottawa, Canadian Institute for Health Information, 2004b.

CIHI. *Inpatient rehabilitation in Canada, 2002–2003*. Ottawa, Canadian Institute for Health Information, 2004c.

CIHI. *National health expenditure trends, 1975–2003*. Ottawa, Canadian Institute for Health Information, 2004d.

CIHI. *Supply, distribution and migration of Canadian physicians, 2003*. Ottawa, Canadian Institute for Health Information, 2004e.

CIHI. *Average payment per physician report, Canada 2002–2003*. Ottawa, Canadian Institute for Health Information, 2004f.

CIHI. *Medical imaging in Canada*. Ottawa, Canadian Institute for Health Information, 2004g.

CIHI. *Drug Expenditure in Canada, 1975-2004*. Ottawa, Canadian Institute for Health Information, 2005.

Clarke JN. *Health, illness, and medicine in Canada: fourth edition*. Toronto, Oxford University Press, 2004.

CMA. *No more time to wait: towards benchmarks and best practices and wait times*. Ottawa, Canadian Medical Association, 2005.

CNA. *The nurse practitioner: CNA position statement*. Ottawa, Canadian Nurses Association, 2003.

College of Nurses of Ontario. *Registered nurses in the extended class*. Toronto, College of Nurses of Ontario, 2004.

Conference Board of Canada. *Fiscal prospects for the federal and provincial/ territorial governments*. Ottawa, Conference Board of Canada, 2004.

Critchley WD. Drug patents and drug prices: the role of the PMPRB. *Address to the Drug Patents Conference, Toronto, 2002*.

CUPE. *Inventory of major privatization initiatives in Canada's health care system, 2003–2004. Ottawa*, Canadian Union of Public Employees, 2004.

Curtis L, Phipps S. Social transfers and the health status of mothers in Norway and Canada. *Social Science and Medicine*, 2004, 58(12):2499–2507.

Deber RB. Delivering health care: public, not-for-profit, or private? In: Marchildon GP, McIntosh T, Forest PG, eds. *The fiscal sustainability of health care in Canada*. Toronto, University of Toronto Press, 2004:233–296.

Decter MB. *Four strong winds: understanding the growing challenges to health care*. Toronto, Stoddard, 2000.

Denis, JL. Governance and management of change in Canada's health system. In: Forest PG, Marchildon GP, McIntosh T, eds. *Changing health care in Canada*. Toronto, University of Toronto Press, 2004:82–114.

Devereaux PJ et al. Payments for care at private-for-profit and private not-for-profit hospitals: a systematic review and meta-analysis. *Canadian Medical Association Journal*, 2004, 170(12):1817–1824.

Epps T, Flood CM. Have we traded away the opportunity for innovative health care reform? The implications of NAFTA for Medicare. *McGill Law Journal*, 2002, 47(4):747–790.

Evans RG, McGrail KM, Morgan SG, Barer ML, Herzman C. Apocalypse no. Population aging and the future of health care systems. *Canadian Journal of Aging*, 2001, 20 (supplement 1):160–191.

Evans RG. *Political wolves and economic sheep. The sustainability of public health insurance in Canada*. Vancouver, Centre for Health Services and Policy Research, University of British Columbia [working paper], 2003.

Evans RG. Financing health care: options, consequences, and objectives. In: Marchildon GP, McIntosh T, Forest PG, eds. *The fiscal sustainability of health care in Canada*. Toronto, University of Toronto Press, 2004:139–196.

Ferris FD, Balfour HM, Bowen K, Farley J, Hardwick M, Lamontagne C, Lundy M, Syme A, West P. *A model to guide hospice palliative care*. Ottawa, Hospice Palliative Care Association, 2002.

Finance Canada. *Fiscal reference tables*. Ottawa, Finance Canada, 2003.

Finance Canada. *Tax expenditures and evaluation*. Ottawa, Finance Canada, 2004.

Flood CM, Archibald T. The illegality of private health care in Canada. *Canadian Medical Association Journal*, 2001, 164(6):825–830.

Foot DK. *Boom, bust and echo: profiting from the demographic shift in the 21st century*. Toronto, Stoddart, 2001.

Giacomini M, Miller F, Browman G. Confronting the "grey zones" of technology assessment: evaluating genetic testing services for public insurance coverage in Canada. *International Journal of Technology Assessment in Health Care*, 2003, 19(2):301–315.

Gorey KM, Holowaty EJ, Fehringer G, Laukkanen E, Moskowitz A, Webster DJ, Richter NL. An international comparison of cancer survival: Toronto, Ontario, and Detroit, Michigan, metropolitan areas. *American Journal of Public Health*, 1997, 87(7):1156–1163.

Gorey KM, Holowaty EJ, Fehringer G, Laukkanen E, Richter NL, Meyer CM. An international comparison of cancer survival: metropolitan Toronto, Ontario, and Honolulu, Hawaii. *American Journal of Public Health*, 2000, 90(12):1866–1872.

Gratzer D. *Code blue: reviving Canada's health care system*. Toronto, ECW Press, 1999.

Gratzer D ed. *Better medicine: reforming Canadian health care*. Toronto, ECW Press, 2002.

Greschner D. How will the Charter of Rights and Freedoms and evolving jurisprudence affect health care costs? In: McIntosh T, Forest PG, Marchildon GP, eds. *The governance of health care in Canada*. Toronto, University of Toronto Press, 2004:83–124.

Grignon M, Paris V, Polton D, with the cooperation of Couffinhal A, Pierrard B. The influence of physician-payment methods on the efficiency of the health care system. In: Forest PG, Marchildon GP, McIntosh T, eds. *Changing health care in Canada*. Toronto, University of Toronto Press, 2004:207–239.

Grishaber-Otto J, Sinclair S. *Bad medicine: trade treaties, privatization and health care reform in Canada*. Ottawa, Canadian Centre for Policy Alternatives, 2004.

Hall, EM. *Canada's national-provincial health program for the 1980s*. Ottawa, National Health and Welfare, 1980.

Hastings JEF. *The community health centre in Canada. Report of the Community Health Centre Project to the Conference of Health Ministers* [JEF Hastings, Chair]. Ottawa, Health and Welfare Canada, 1972.

Health Canada. *Programmatic guidelines for screening for cancer of the cervix.* Ottawa, Quality Management Working Group, Cervical Cancer Prevention Network, 1998.

Health Canada. *A report on mental illnesses in Canada.* Ottawa, Health Canada, 2002.

Health Canada. *Learning from SARS: renewal of public health.* A report of the National Advisory Committee on SARS and Public Health [D Naylor, Chair]. Ottawa, Health Canada, 2003a.

Health Canada. *Annual report on First Nations and Inuit control, 2001/2002.* Ottawa, Health Canada, 2003b.

Health Canada. *Complementary and alternative health care: the other mainstream?* Ottawa, Health Canada, 2003c (Health Policy Research, issue 7, November 2003).

Health Canada. *Canada Health Act annual report, 2003–2004.* Ottawa, Health Canada, 2004.

Health Charities Council of Canada. *Partners for improvement. Observations and recommendations from the Health Charities Council of Canada. A brief to the Commission on the Future of Health Care in Canada.* Ottawa, Health Charities Council of Canada, 2001.

Health Council of Canada. *Health care renewal in Canada: accelerating change.* Toronto, Health Council of Canada, 2005.

Healy J, McKee M. The role and function of hospitals. In: McKee M and Healy J. eds. *Hospitals in a changing Europe.* Buckingham, Open University Press, 2002.

Hilless M, Healy J. *Health care systems in transition: Australia.* Copenhagen, WHO Regional Office for Europe on behalf of the European Observatory on Health Care Systems and Policies, 2001.

Hjortsberg C, Ghatnekar O. *Health care systems in transition: Sweden.* Copenhagen, WHO Regional Office for Europe on behalf of the European Observatory on Health Care Systems and Policies, 2001.

Houston, CS. *Steps on the road to Medicare: why Saskatchewan led the way.* Montreal and Kingston, McGill-Queen's University Press, 2002.

Hurley J. Regionalization and the allocation of healthcare resources to meet population health needs. *Healthcare Papers*, 2004, 5:34–39.

Hussey P, Anderson GF. A comparison of single- and multi-payer health insurance systems and options for reform. *Health Policy*, 2003, 66:215–228.

Hussey PS et al. US health care spending in an international context: why is US spending so high and can we afford it? *Health Affairs,* 2004, 23(3):10–25.

Hutchison B, Abelson J, Lavis J. Primary care in Canada: So much innovation, so little change. *Health Affairs,* 2001, 20(3):116–131.

IMS HEALTH Canada. IMS HEALTH Canada Drug Monitor. Mississauga, ON, IMS HEALTH Canada Inc., 2004 (www.imshealthcanada.com).

Jackman M. Section 7 of the Charter and health-care spending. In: Marchildon GP, McIntosh T, Forest PG, eds. *The fiscal sustainability of health care in Canada.* Toronto, University of Toronto Press, 2004:110–136.

Johnson AW. *Dream no little dreams. A biography of the Douglas government in Saskatchewan.* Toronto, University of Toronto Press, 2004a.

Johnson JR. International trade agreements and Canadian health care. In: Marchildon GP, McIntosh T, Forest PG, eds. *The fiscal sustainability of health care in Canada.* Toronto, University of Toronto Press, 2004b:369–402.

Jonas WB, Levin JS, eds. *Essentials of complementary and alternative medicine.* Philadephia, Lippincott, Williams & Wilkins, 1999.

Kapur A. Global solidarity against globalized tobacco: The world's first modern health treaty. *Canadian Medical Association Journal,* 2003, 168(10):1263–1264.

Katzmarzyk PT. The Canadian obesity epidemic, 1985–1998. *Canadian Medical Association Journal,* 2002, 166(8):1039–1040.

Katzmarzyk PT, Ardern CI. Overweight and obesity mortality trends in Canada, 1985–2000. *Canadian Journal of Public Health,* 2004, 95(1):16–20.

Kelner M, Wellman B, Boon H, Welsh S. Responses of established healthcare to the professions of CAM in Ontario. *Social Science and Medicine,* 2004, 59(5):915–930.

Laporte A, Ferguson B. Income inequality and mortality: time series evidence from Canada. *Health Policy,* 2003, 66:107–111.

Lavoie JG. Governed by contracts: the development of indigenous primary health services in Canada, Australia and New Zealand. *Journal of Aboriginal Health,* 2004, 1(1):6–24.

Lazar H, St-Hilaire F, eds. *Money, politics and health care: reconstructing the federal-provincial partnership.* Montreal, Institute for Research on Public Policy, 2004.

Lazar H, St-Hilaire F, Tremblay JF. Federal health care funding: Toward a new fiscal pact. In: Lazar H, St-Hillaire F, eds. *Money, politics and health care: reconstructing the federal-provincial partnership.* Montreal, Institute for Research on Public Policy, 2004.

Leeson H. Constitutional jurisdiction over health and health care services in Canada. In: *The governance of health care in Canada*. Toronto, University of Toronto Press, 2004:50–82.

Lemchuk-Favel L, Jock JG. Aboriginal health systems in Canada: nine case studies. *Journal of Aboriginal Health*, 2004, 1(1):6–24.

Lewis S, Kouri D. Regionalization: making sense of the Canadian experience. *HealthcarePapers*, 2004, 5(1):12–31.

Lexchin J. Pharmaceuticals, patents and politics: Canada and Bill C-22. *International Journal of Health Services*, 1993, 23(1):147–160.

Lomas J. Devolving authority for health care in Canada's provinces: 4. Emerging issues and prospects. *Canadian Medical Association Journal*, 1997, 156(6):817–823.

Mackenzie H. *Financing Canada's hospitals: public alternatives to P3s*. Toronto, Hugh Mackenzie and Associates, 2004.

Maioni A. *Parting at the crossroads: the emergence of health insurance in the United States and Canada*. Princeton, NJ, Princeton University Press, 1998.

Maioni A. Roles and responsibilities in health care policy. In: McIntosh T, Forest PG, Marchildon, GP eds. *The governance of health care in Canada*. Toronto, University of Toronto Press, 2004:169–198.

Makomaski-Illing EM, Kaiserman MJ. Mortality attributable to tobacco use in Canada and its regions, 1994 and 1996. *Chronic Diseases in Canada*, 1999, 20(3):111–117.

Marchildon GP. Fin de siècle Canada: The federal government in retreat. In: McCarthy P, Jones P, eds. *Distintegration or transformation: the crisis of the state in advanced industrial societies*. New York, St. Martin's Press, 1995:133–151.

Marchildon GP. The many worlds of fiscal sustainability. Introduction. In: Marchildon GP, McIntosh, T, Forest PG, eds. *The fiscal sustainability of health care in Canada*. Toronto, University of Toronto Press, 2004a:3–23.

Marchildon GP. *Three choices for the future of Medicare*. Toronto, Caledon Institute of Social Policy, 2004b.

Marchildon GP. The public/private debate in the funding, administration and delivery of healthcare in Canada. *Healthcare Papers*, 2004c, 4(4):61–68.

Marchildon GP. Canadian health system reforms: lessons for Australia? *Australian Health Review*, 2005, 29(1):105–119.

Marriott J, Mable AL. Integrated models: international trends and implications for Canada. In: *Striking a balance: health care systems in Canada and elsewhere*. Ottawa, National Forum on Health, 1998:551–672.

Martin CM, Hogg WE. How family physicians are funded in Canada. *Medical Journal of Australia*, 2004, 181(2):111–112.

Mathers CD et al. *Estimates of DALE for 191 countries: methods and results.* Geneva, World Health Organization, Global Programme on Health Policy, 2000 (working paper No. 16).

Maxwell J et al. *Citizens' dialogue on the future of health care in Canada.* Report prepared for the Commission on the Future of Health Care in Canada. Ottawa, Canadian Policy Research Networks, 2002.

Maxwell J, Rosell S, Forest PG. Giving citizens a voice in healthcare policy in Canada. *British Medical Journal*, 2003, 326:1031–1033.

McDaid D. Co-ordinating health technology assessment in Canada: a European perspective. *Health Policy,* 2003, 63:205–213.

McDonnell TE, McDonnell DE. Policy forum: taxing for health care – the Ontario model, 2004. *Canadian Tax Journal*, 2005, 53(1):107–134.

McFarlane L, Prado C. *The best-laid plans: health care's problems and prospects.* Montreal, McGill-Queen's University Press, 2002.

McGrail KM, Evans RG, Barer ML, Sheps SB, Hertzman C, Kazanjian A. The quick and the dead: "managing" inpatient care in British Columbia hospitals, 1969 to 1995/96. *Health Services Research*, 2001, 35(6):1319–1338.

McIntosh T. Intergovernmental relations, social policy and federal transfers after Romanow. *Canadian Public Administration,* 2004, 47(1):27–51.

McKay L. *Making the Lalonde report.* Ottawa, Canadian Policy Research Networks, 2001.

McKillop I. Financial rules as a catalyst for change in the Canadian health care system. In: Forest PG, Marchildon GP, McIntosh T, eds. *Changing health care in Canada.* Toronto, University of Toronto Press, 2004:54–81.

McKillop I, Pink GH, Johnson L. *The financial management of acute care in Canada: a review of funding, performance monitoring and reporting practices.* Ottawa, Canadian Institute for Health Information, 2001.

Mendelsohn M. *Canadians' thoughts on their health care system: preserving the Canadian model through innovation.* Saskatoon, Commission on the Future of Health Care in Canada, 2002.

Menon D. Pharmaceutical cost control in Canada: Does it work? *Health Affairs,* 2001, 20(3):92–103.

Mhatre SL, Deber RB. From equal access to health care to equitable access to health: a review of Canadian provincial health commissions and reports. *International Journal of Health Services*, 1992, 22(4):645–68.

Mintzes B, Barer ML, Kravitz RL, Kazanjian A, Bassett K, Lexchin J, Evans RG, Pan R, Marion SA. Influence of direct to consumer advertising and patients' requests on prescribing decisions: two site cross sectional survey. *British Medical Journal*, 2002, 324:278–279.

Mohr J. American medical malpractice litigation in historical perspective. *JAMA*, 2000, 283(13):1731–1737.

Morgan S. Sources of variation in provincial drug spending. *Canadian Medical Association Journal*, 2004, 170(3):329–330.

Morgan S. Canadian prescription drug costs surpass $18 billion. *Canadian Medical Association Journal*, 2005, 172(10):1323–1324.

Morgan S, Hurley J. Technological change as a cost-driver in health care. In: Marchildon, GP, McIntosh T, Forest PG, eds. *The fiscal sustainability of health care in Canada*. Toronto, University of Toronto Press, 2004:27–50.

Mossialos E, Dixon A. Funding health care: an introduction. In: Mossialos E et al, eds. *Funding health care: options for Europe*. Buckingham, Open University Press, 2002:1–30.

Mossialos E, Thompson S. *Voluntary health insurance in the European Union*. Brussels, World Health Organization on behalf of the European Observatory on Health Systems and Policies, 2004.

National Advisory Committee on Immunization. *Canadian immunization guide, fifth edition*. Ottawa, Health Canada, Cat. H49-8/1998E, 1998.

National Steering Committee on Patient Safety. *Building a safer system: a national integrated strategy for improving patient safety in Canadian health care*. Ottawa, National Steering Committee on Patient Safety, 2002.

Naylor CD. *Private practice, public payment: Canadian medicine and the politics of health insurance, 1911–1966*. Montreal and Kingston, McGill-Queen's University Press, 1986.

Nolte E, McKee M. Measuring the health of nations: analysis of mortality amenable to health care. *British Medical Journal*, 2003, 327:1129–1134.

Noseworthy TW, McGurran JJ, Hadorn DC and the Steering Committee of the Western Canada Waiting List Project. Waiting for scheduled services in Canada: development of priority-setting scoring systems. *Journal of Evaluation in Clinical Practice*, 2003, 9(1):23–31.

Nova Scotia. *The report of the Nova Scotia Royal Commission on Health Care. Towards a new strategy*. Halifax, Queen's Printer, 1989.

O'Brien-Pallas L. Where to from here? *Canadian Journal of Nursing Research*, 2002, 33(4):3–14.

OECD. *Creating rural indicators for shaping territorial policies.* Paris, Organisation for Economic Co-operation and Development, 1994.

OECD. *Health at a glance.* Paris, Organisation for Economic Co-operation and Development, 2001.

OECD. OECD in figures. Statistics on the member countries. *OECD Observer 2003.* Supplement number 1. Paris, Organisation for Economic Co-operation and Development, 2003.

OECD. *OECD health data 2004: a comparative analysis of 30 countries, fourth edition.* Paris, Organisation for Economic Co-operation and Development, 2004a.

OECD. *Part II to IV of national accounts of OECD countries, Vol. 1.* Paris, Organisation for Economic Co-operation and Development, 2004b.

Ontario. *Final report of the Task Force on the Use and Provision of Medical Services.* Toronto, Task Force on the Use and Provision of Medical Services, 1990.

Ontario. *Weighing the balance: a review of the regulated Health Professions Act.* Toronto, Health Professions Advisory Committee for the Government of Ontario, 1999.

Ontario. *Looking backward, looking forward,* 2 volumes [D. Sinclair, Chair]. Toronto, Health Services Restructuring Committee, 2000.

Ontario. Ontario report to premiers. Genetics and gene patenting: charting new territories in healthcare. Toronto, Government of Ontario, 2002.

Ontario. Ontario Family Health Network transition. Government of Ontario, 2004 (http://www.ontariofamilyhealthnetwork.gov.on.ca/english/, accessed on 1 October 2004).

Ontario. *Report on the integration of primary health care nurse practitioners into the province of Ontario: final report, revised January 2005.* Toronto, Government of Ontario, 2005.

O'Reilly P. The federal/provincial/territorial health conference system. In Adams D, ed. *Federalism, democracy and health policy in Canada.* Montreal and Kingston, McGill-Queen's University Press, 2001.

Ouellet R. The effects of international trade agreements and options for upcoming negotiations. In: Marchildon GP, McIntosh T, Forest PG. eds. *The fiscal sustainability of health care in Canada.* Toronto, University of Toronto Press, 2004:403–422.

Palmer D'Angelo Consulting Inc. *Impact study of a national pharmacare program for Canada: an update to the 1997 report.* Ottawa, Palmer D'Angelo Consulting Inc., 2002.

Phillips K, Swan WR. *Health care systems in transition: Canada (preliminary version)*. Copenhagen, WHO Regional Office for Europe, 1996.

PMPRB. *Patented Medicine Prices Review Board annual report 2003*. Ottawa, Patented Medicine Prices Review Board, 2004.

Pritchard JR. *Liability and compensation in health care*. Toronto, University of Toronto Press, 1990.

Quebec. *Rapport de la Commission d'enquête sur les service de santé et les services sociaux* [J Rochon, Chair]. Quebec, Commission d'enquête sur les services de santé et les services sociaux, 1988.

Quebec. *Emerging solutions: report and recommendations* [M Clair, Chair]. Quebec, Commission d'étude sur les services de santé et les services sociaux, 2002.

Quebec. *Pour un régime d'assurance médicaments équitable et viable. Rapport préparé par le Comité sur la pertinence et la faisabilité d'un régime universel public d'assurance médicaments au Québec* [C Montmarquette, Président]. Quebec, Ministère de la Santé et des Services Sociaux, 2001.

Ramsay C. Determining the extent of public financing of programs and services. In: Marchildon GP, McIntosh T, Forest PG., eds. *The fiscal sustainability of health care in Canada*. Toronto, University of Toronto Press, 2004:197–232.

Reichert B, Windover M. Canadian pharma … falling behind? *Biotechnology Focus*, 2002, 5(3):16–18.

Robinson R, Dixon A. *Health care systems in transition: United Kingdom*. Copenhagen, WHO Regional Office for Europe on behalf of the European Observatory on Health Systems and Policies, 1999.

Rock G. Changes in the Canadian blood system: the Krever Inquiry, Canadian Blood Services and Héma-Quebec. *Transfusion Science*, 2000, 22:29–37.

Roehrig C, Kargus K. Health technology assessment in Canada and the G7 countries: a comparative analysis of the role of HTA agencies in the decision-making process. Ottawa, Health Canada, Health Care System Division working paper, November 2003.

Romanow RJ and Marchildon GP. Psychological services and the future of health care in Canada. *Canadian Psychology*, 2003, 44(3):283–298.

Rubin RJ, Mendelson D. A framework for cost-sharing policy analysis. *Pharmacoeconomics*, 1996, 10 (Supplement 2):56–67.

Sandier S, Paris V, Polton D. *Health care systems in transition: France*. Copenhagen, WHO Regional Office for Europe on behalf of the European Observatory on Health Systems and Policies, 2004.

Sanger M, Sinclair S. *Putting health first: Canadian health care reform in a globalizing world.* Ottawa, Canadian Centre for Policy Alternatives, 2004.

Saskatchewan. *Future directions for health care in Saskatchewan* [D Murray, Chair]. Regina, Saskatchewan Commission on Directions in Health Care, 1990.

Saskatchewan. *Caring for Medicare: sustaining a quality system* [KJ Fyke, Commissioner]. Regina, Saskatchewan Commission on Medicare, 2001.

Senate. *Quality end-of-life care: the rights of every Canadian. Final report* [S Carstairs, Chair]. Ottawa, Standing Senate Committee on Social Affairs, Science and Technology, 2000.

Senate. *The health of Canadians – the federal role. Volume one. The story so far* [MJL Kirby, Chair]. Ottawa, Standing Senate Committee on Social Affairs, Science and Technology, 2001a.

Senate. *The health of Canadians – the federal role. Volume four. Issues and options* [MJL Kirby, Chair]. Ottawa, Standing Senate Committee on Social Affairs, Science and Technology, 2001b.

Senate. *The health of Canadians – the federal role. Final report on the state of the health care system in Canada. Volume six. Recommendations for reform* [MJL Kirby, Chair]. Ottawa, Standing Senate Committee on Social Affairs, Science and Technology, 2002a.

Senate. *The health of Canadians – the federal role. Current trends and challenges. Volume two. Current trends and future challenges* [MJL Kirby, Chair]. Ottawa, Standing Senate Committee on Social Affairs, Science and Technology, 2002b.

Senate. *The health of Canadians – the federal role. Volume three. Health care systems in other countries* [MJL Kirby, Chair]. Ottawa, Standing Senate Committee on Social Affairs, Science and Technology, 2002c.

Senate. *The health of Canadians – the federal role. Volume five. Principles and recommendations for reform – Part 1* [MJL Kirby, Chair]. Ottawa, Standing Senate Committee on Social Affairs, Science and Technology, 2002d.

Shushelski C. Patients' bill of rights. *Hospital Quarterly,* 1999, 3(1):50–53.

Starfield B. Summing up: primary health care reform in contemporary health care systems. In: Wilson R, Short SED, Dorland J, eds. *Implementing primary care reform: barriers and facilitators.* Kingston, ON, McGill-Queen's University Press for School of Policy Studies, Queen's University, 2004:151–164.

Statistics Canada. *2001 census of population.* Ottawa, Statistics Canada, 2001a.

Statistics Canada. *Canadian community health survey, 2000/01.* Ottawa, Statistics Canada, 2001b.

Statistics Canada. *Canada food stats,* 2:2. Ottawa, Statistics Canada, 2002.

Statistics Canada. *Health indicators.* 2: November 2003. Ottawa, Statistics Canada, 2003.

Statistics Canada. *1975 to 2004 national accounts.* Ottawa, Statistics Canada, 2004.

Statistics Canada. *Health indicators,* 2: June 2005. Ottawa, Statistics Canada, 2005.

Statistics Canada. CANSIM II, various tables. Ottawa, Statistics Canada.

Statistics Canada. *The Daily.* Ottawa, Statistics Canada, various dates.

Stephens T et al. School-based smoking cessation: economic costs versus benefits. *Chronic Diseases in Canada,* 2000, 21(2):62–67.

Sullivan T, Dobrow M, Thompson L, Hudson A. Reconstructing cancer services in Ontario. *Healthcare Papers,* 2004, 5:69–80.

Sussex J. *The economics of the Private Finance Initiatives in the NHS.* London, Office of Health Economics, 2001.

Sutherland LP, Verhoef MJ. Why do patients seek a second opinion or alternative medicine? *Journal of Clinical Gastroenterology,* 1994, 19(3):194–197.

Taylor M. *Health insurance and Canadian public policy: the seven decisions that created the Canadian healthcare system, second edition.* Montreal, McGill-Queens University Press, 1987.

Tully P, Saint-Pierre E. Downsizing Canada's hospitals, 1986/87 to 1994/95. Statistics Canada *Health Reports,* Spring 1997, 8(4):33–39.

Tuohy CH. *Accidental logics: the dynamics of change in the health care arena in the United States, Britain, and Canada.* New York, Oxford University Press, 1999.

Tuohy CH. The costs of constraint and prospects for health care reform in Canada. *Health Affairs,* 2002, 21(3):32–46.

Tuohy CH. Health care reform strategies in cross-national context: implications for primary care in Ontario. In: Wilson R et al, eds. *Implementing primary care reform: barriers and facilitators.* Montreal and Kingston, McGill-Queen's University Press, 2004.

Waldram JB, Herring DA, Young DK. *Aboriginal health in Canada: historical, cultural and epidemiological perspectives.* Toronto, University of Toronto Press, 1995.

Welsh S, Kelner M, Wellman B, Boon H. Moving forward? Complementary and alternative practitioners seeking self-regulation. *Sociology of Health and Illness*, 2004, 26(2):216–241.

WHO. *The world health report 2000. Health systems: improving performance.* Geneva, World Health Organization, 2000.

WHO. *The world health report 2001. Mental health: new understanding, new hope.* Geneva, World Health Organization, 2001.

Wiktorowicz M, Lapp M, Brodie I, Abelson D. Nonprofit groups and health policy in Ontario: Assessing strategies and influence in a changing environment. In: Brock KL, ed. *Delicate dances: public policy and the nonprofit sector.* Kingston, ON, McGill-Queen's University Press for School of Policy Studies, Queen's University, 2003:171–219.

Wilson K, McCrea-Logie J, Lazar H. Understanding the impact of intergovernmental relations on public health. Lessons from reform initiatives in the blood system and health surveillance. *Canadian Public Policy,* 2004, 30(2):177–194.

Wilson R, Shortt SED, Dorland J, eds. *Implementing primary care reform: barriers and facilitators.* Kingston, ON, McGill-Queen's University Press for School of Policy Studies, Queen's University, 2004.

Wolfson S. Use of paraprofessionals: the Saskatchewan Dental Plan. In: Glor E, ed. *Policy innovation in the Saskatchewan public sector.* Toronto, Captus Press, 1997.

Woolhandler S, Campbell T, Himmelstein DU. Costs of health care administration in the United States and Canada. *New England Journal of Medicine,* 2003, 349(8):768–775.

Yalnizyan A. *Paul Martin's permanent revolution.* Ottawa, Canadian Centre for Policy Alternatives, 2004a.

Yalnizyan A. Accepting the Pharmacare prescription. *Canadian Healthcare Manager,* September 2004b.

Zboril-Benson L. Why nurses are calling in sick: the impact of health-care restructuring. *Canadian Journal of Nursing Research,* 2002, 33(4):89–108.

11. Useful websites

1. Federal government

Health Canada: http://www.hc-sc.gc.ca

Health Canada, First Nations and Inuit health branch: http://www.hc-sc.gc.ca/fnihb-dgspni/fnihb

Statistics Canada: http://www.statcan.ca

2. Provincial and territorial health ministries

Alberta, Alberta Health and Wellness: http://www.health.gov.ab.ca

British Columbia, Ministry of Health Services: http://www.gov.bc.ca/bvprd/bc/channel.do?action=ministry&channelID=-8387&navId=NAV_ID_province

Manitoba, Manitoba Health: http://www.gov.mb.ca/health

New Brunswick, Health and Wellness: http://www.gnb.ca/0051/index-e.asp

Newfoundland and Labrador, Health and Community Services: http://public.gov.nf.ca/health

Northwest Territories, Health and Social Services: http://www.hlthss.gov.nt.ca

Nova Scotia, Department of Health: http://www.gov.ns.ca/heal

Nunavut, Health and Social Services: http://www.gov.nu.ca/hsssite/hssmain.shtml

Ontario, Ministry of Health and Long-Term Care: http://www.health.gov.on.ca

Prince Edward Island, Health and Social Services: http://www.gov.pe.ca/hss

Quebec, Santé et Services sociaux: http://www.msss.gouv.qc.ca

Saskatchewan, Saskatchewan Health: http://www.health.gov.sk.ca

Yukon Territories, Department of Health and Social Services: http://www.hss.gov.yk.ca

3. National and intergovernmental agencies

Canada Health Infoway: http://www.canadahealthinfoway.com

Canadian Blood Services: http://www.bloodservices.ca

Canadian Coordinating Office for Health Technology Assessment: http://www.ccohta.ca

Canadian Institute for Health Information (CIHI): http://cihi.ca

Health Council of Canada: http://hcc-ccs.com

Patented Medicine Prices Review Board: http://www.pmprb-cepmb.gc.ca

Public Health Agency of Canada: http://www.phac-aspc.gc.ca

4. Provincial health agencies of note

Alberta Heritage Foundation for Medical Research: http://www.ahfmr.ab.ca

CardiacCare Network of Ontario: http://www.ccn.on.ca

Collège des médicins du Québec: http://www.cmq.org

Institute for Clinical Evaluative Sciences: http://www.ices.on.ca

Manitoba Centre for Health Policy: http://www.umanitoba.ca/centres/mchp

Ontario Hospital Association: http://www.oha.com

Quebec, Agence d'évaluation des technologies et des modes d'intervention en santé: http://www.aetmis.gouv.qc.ca

Quebec , Héma-Québec: http://www.hema-Quebec .qc.ca

Quebec , La Régie de l'assurance maladie du Quebec: http://www.ramq.gouv.qc.ca/

Saskatchewan, Health Quality Council: http://www.hqc.sk.ca

Saskatchewan Health Research Foundation: http://www.shrf.ca

5. National non-profit and provider organizations

Alzheimer Society of Canada: http://www.alzheimer.ca

Association of Canadian Academic Healthcare Organizations: http://www.acaho.org

Association of Workers' Compensation Boards of Canada: http://www.awcbc.
org

Asthma Society of Canada: http://www.asthma.ca

Canadian Breast Cancer Network: http://www.cbcn.ca

Canadian Cystic Fibrosis Foundation: http://www.ccff.ca

Canada's Research-Based Pharmaceuticals Companies: http://www.
canadapharma.org

Canadian AIDS Society: http://www.cdnaids.ca

Canadian Association for Community Care: http://www.cacc-acssc.com

Canadian Association of Medical Radiation Technologists: http://www.camrt.
ca

Canadian Association of Occupational Therapists: http://www.caot.ca

Canadian Association of Retired Persons: http://www.50plus.com

Canadian Cancer Society: http://www.cancer.ca

Canadian Chiropractic Association: http://www.ccachiro.org

Canadian Council on Health Services Accreditation: http://www.cchsa.ca

Canadian Dental Association: http://www.cda-adc.ca

Canadian Diabetes Association: http://www.diabetes.ca

Canadian Generic Pharmaceutical Association: http://www.cdma-acfpp.org

Canadian Health Coalition: http://www.healthcoalition.ca

Canadian Healthcare Association: http://www.cha.ca

Canadian Hemophilia Society: http://www.hemophilia.ca

Canadian Homecare Association: http://www.cdnhomecare.on.ca

Canadian Hospice Palliative Care Association: http://www.chpca.net

Canadian Lung Association: http://www.lung.ca

Canadian Medical Foundation: http://www.medicalfoundation.ca

Canadian Organization for Rare Disorders: http://www.cord.ca

Canadian Mental Health Association: http://www.cmha.ca

Canadian National Institute for the Blind: http://www.cnib.ca

Canadian Pharmacists Association: http://www.pharmacists.ca

Canadian Physiotherapy Association: http://www.physiotherapy.ca

Canadian Psychological Association: http://www.cpa.ca/

Canadian Public Health Association: http://www.cpha.ca/

Canadian Society for Medical Laboratory Science: http://www.csmls.org

Canadian Women's Health Network: http://www.cwhn.ca

College of Family Physicians of Canada: http://www.cfpc.ca

Epilepsy Canada: http://www.epilepsy.ca

Health Charities Coalition of Canada: http://www.healthcharities.ca

Heart and Stroke Foundation of Canada: http://ww2.heartandstroke.ca

Hepatitis C Society of Canada: http://www.hepatitiscsociety.com

Huntington Society of Canada: http://www.hsc-ca.org

Medical Council of Canada: http://www.mcc.ca

Multiple Sclerosis Society of Canada: http://www.mssociety.ca

Muscular Dystrophy Association of Canada: http://www.mdac.ca

National Aboriginal Health Organization: http://www.naho.ca

National Network for Mental Health: http://www.nnmh.ca

Osteoporosis Society of Canada: http://www.osteoporosis.ca

Parkinson Society Canada: http://www.parkinson.ca

Royal College of Dentists of Canada: http://www.rcdc.ca

The Arthritis Society: http://www.arthritis.ca

The Canadian Association of Naturopathic Doctors: http://www.
naturopathicassoc.ca

The Canadian Life and Health Insurance Association: http://www.clhia.ca

The Canadian Medical Association: http://www.cma.ca

The Canadian Nurses Association: http://www.cna-nurses.ca/cna

The Kidney Foundation of Canada: http://www.kidney.ca

The Royal College of Physicians and Surgeons of Canada: http://rcpsc.medical.
org

6. Health policy and research

Atlantic Health Promotion Research Centre: http://www.ahprc.dal.ca

Canadian Association for Health Services and Policy Research: http://www.
cahspr.ca

Canadian Centre for Analysis of Regionalization and Health: http://www.
regionalization.org

Canadian Consortium for Health Promotion Research: http://www.utoronto.
ca/chp/CCHPR

Canadian Health Services Research Foundation: http://www.chsrf.ca/index.
php

Canadian Institute of Child Health: http://www.cich.ca

Canadian Institutes of Health Research: http://www.cihr-irsc.gc.ca

Canadian Policy Research Networks, Health Network: http://www.cprn.org

Centre for Addiction and Mental Health: http://www.camh.net

Centre for Evidence-Based Medicine: http://www.cebm.utoronto.ca

Centre for Health Economics and Policy Analysis: http://www.chepa.org

Centre for Health Evidence: http://www.cche.net

Centre for Health Services and Policy Research: http://www.chspr.ubc.ca

Centre for Health Promotion: http://www.utoronto.ca/chp

Centre for Health Promotion Studies: http://www.chps.ualberta.ca

Centre for Research in Women's Health: http://www.crwh.org

Centre for Rural and Northern Health Research: http://cranhr.laurentian.ca

Centres of Excellence for Women's Health: http://www.cewh-cesf.ca

Dalhousie University, Population Health Research Unit: http://phru.medicine.dal.ca

Genome Canada: http://www.genomecanada.ca

Health Law Institute: http://www.law.ualberta.ca/centres/hli

Institute for Work and Health: http://www.iwh.on.ca

Institute of Health Economics: http://www.ihe.ab.ca

Institute of Health Promotion Research: http://www.ihpr.ubc.ca

McMaster University, Health Information Research Unit: http://hiru.mcmaster.ca

National Network on Environments and Women's Health: http://www.yorku.ca/nnewh

Population Health Research Institute: http://www.phri.ca

Queen's University, The Centre for Health Services and Policy Research: http://chspr.queensu.ca

7. Recent health reports

Alberta, Premier's Advisory Council on Health for Alberta: http://www.premiersadvisory.com

Commission on the Future of Health Care in Canada: http://www.hc-sc.gc.ca/english/care/romanow

National Advisory Committee on SARS and Public Health: http://www.hc-sc.gc.ca/english/protection/warnings/sars/learning

National Forum on Health: http://www.hc-sc.gc.ca/english/care/health_forum/
forum_e.htm

Ontario, The Health Services Restructuring Commission: http://www.health.
gov.on.ca/hsrc/home.htm

Quebec , Commission d'étude sur les services de santé et les services sociaux:
http://www.msss.gouv.qc.ca/en/documentation/publications.html

Saskatchewan, Commission on Medicare: http://www.health.gov.sk.ca/mc_dp_
commission_on_medicare-bw.pdf

Standing Senate Committee on Social Affairs, Science and Technology, health
reports: http://www.parl.gc.ca/37/2/parlbus/commbus/senate/com-e/soci-e/rep-
e/repoct02vol6-e.htm

http://www.parl.gc.ca/37/1/parlbus/commbus/senate/com-e/soci-e/rep-e/
repapr02vol5-e.htm

http://www.parl.gc.ca/37/1/parlbus/commbus/senate/com-e/soci-e/rep-e/
repintsep01-e.htm

http://www.parl.gc.ca/37/1/parlbus/commbus/senate/com-e/soci-e/rep-e/
repjan01vol3-e.htm

http://www.parl.gc.ca/37/1/parlbus/commbus/senate/com-e/soci-e/rep-e/
repjan01vol2-e.htm

http://www.parl.gc.ca/37/1/parlbus/commbus/senate/com-e/soci-e/rep-e/
repintmar01-e.htm

The Health Systems in Transition profiles

A series of the European Observatory on Health Systems and Policies

The Health Systems in Transition (HiT) country profiles provide an analytical description of each health care system and of reform initiatives in progress or under development. They aim to provide relevant comparative information to support policy-makers and analysts in the development of health care systems and reforms in the countries of the European Region and beyond. The HiT profiles are building blocks that can be used:

- to learn in detail about different approaches to the financing, organization and delivery of health care services;
- to describe accurately the process, content and implementation of health care reform programmes;
- to highlight common challenges and areas that require more in-depth analysis; and
- to provide a tool for the dissemination of information on health systems and the exchange of experiences of reform strategies between policy-makers and analysts in countries of the WHO European Region.

How to obtain a HiT

All HiT profiles are available in PDF format on *www.observatory.dk*, where you can also join our listserve for monthly updates of the activities of the European Observatory on Health Systems and Policies, including new HiTs, books in our co-published series with Open University Press (English), policy briefs, the *EuroObserver* newsletter and the *EuroHealth* journal. If you would like to order a paper copy of a HiT, please write to:

The publications of the European Observatory on Health Systems and Policies are available on www.euro.who.int/observatory

info@obs.euro.who.int

HiT country profiles published to date:

Albania (1999, 2002[a,g])
Andorra (2004)
Armenia (2001[g])
Australia (2002)
Austria (2001[e])
Azerbaijan (2004)
Belgium (2000)
Bosnia and Herzegovina (2002[g])
Bulgaria (1999, 2003[b])
Canada (2005)
Croatia (1999)
Cyprus (2004)
Czech Republic (2000, 2005)
Denmark (2001)
Estonia (2000, 2004)
Finland (2002)
France (2004[c])
Georgia (2002[d,g])
Germany (2000[e], 2004[e])
Hungary (1999, 2004)
Iceland (2003)
Israel (2003)
Italy (2001)
Kazakhstan (1999[g])
Kyrgyzstan (2000[g])
Latvia (2001)
Lithuania (2000)
Luxembourg (1999)
Malta (1999)
Netherlands (2004)
New Zealand (2002)
Norway (2000)
Poland (1999)
Portugal (1999, 2004)
Republic of Moldova (2002[g])
Romania (2000[f])
Russian Federation (2003[g])
Slovakia (2000, 2004)
Slovenia (2002)
Spain (2000[h])
Sweden (2001)
Switzerland (2000)
Tajikistan (2000)
The former Yugoslav Republic of Macedonia (2000)
Turkey (2002[g,i])
Turkmenistan (2000)
Ukraine (2004[g])
United Kingdom of Great Britain and Northern Ireland (1999[g])
Uzbekistan (2001[g])

Key

All HiTs are available in English.
When noted, they are also available
in other languages:

[a] Albanian
[b] Bulgarian
[c] French
[d] Georgian
[e] German
[f] Romanian
[g] Russian
[h] Spanish
[i] Turkish